HIPPOCRATES

from a head recently discovered near Rome and now in
the Ostia Museum.

Photograph by kind permission of G. Becatti.

The Greek inscription on the base reads:

'Short is life, but long is the age we mortals spend
below the ground; it is the lot of all to bear the fate,
whatever it be, that god apportions.'

The first words are a reminiscence of *Aphorisms* I, 1.

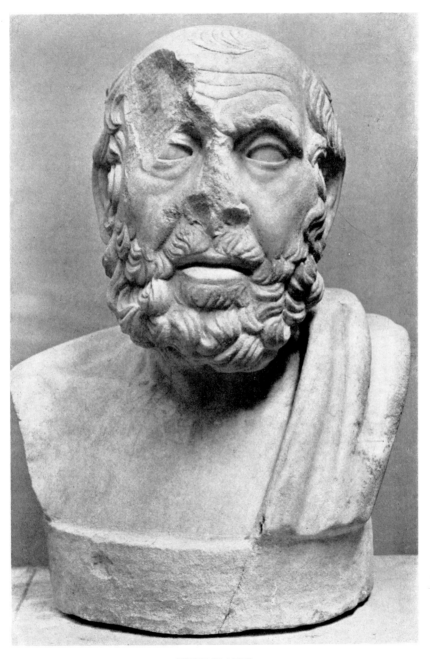

HIPPOCRATES
from a head recently discovered near Rome and now in the Ostia Museum.
Photograph by kind permission of G. Becatti.

The Medical Works of
HIPPOCRATES

*A new translation from the original Greek made
especially for English readers by the collaboration of*

JOHN CHADWICK, M.A. (Cantab.)
sometime Scholar of Corpus Christi College, Cambridge

and

W. N. MANN, M.D. (Lond.), F.R.C.P.
Assistant Physician to Guy's Hospital

BLACKWELL
SCIENTIFIC PUBLICATIONS
OXFORD

Published simultaneously in the United States of America by Charles C Thomas, Publisher, 301-327 East Lawrence Avenue, Springfield, Illinois.

Published simultaneously in Canada by The Ryerson Press, Queen Street West, Toronto 2.

First printed, December, 1950

Printed in Great Britain for BLACKWELL SCIENTIFIC PUBLICATIONS, LTD. by A. R. MOWBRAY & Co. LIMITED, London and Oxford

PREFACE

IN presenting to the public a new translation of the works of Hippocrates, we are aware that we follow a long line of editors and scholars who have laboured to make available to students of medicine throughout the centuries the writings of the foremost physician of antiquity. Paradoxically, during the last century, which has seen the greatest advance in medical learning since Greek days, the work of Hippocrates has been less generally known to the student than at any other time. The most famous and almost only complete edition, that of Littré with French translation in ten volumes, is now only to be found in a few libraries. Of English translations that of F. Adams was published a century ago; and there remains the scholarly text and translation in the Loeb Library by W. H. S. Jones and E. T. Withington. Our object in presenting this small volume is to enable the medical student or doctor, and indeed all who are interested in the beginnings of science, to gain a first-hand acquaintance with early Greek medicine. The translation is therefore designed for the reader who has no Greek and we have endeavoured to reproduce faithfully the thoughts, comments and observations recorded in antiquity. We believe it important that the many great truths embodied in this work should remain a part of the armamentarium of the physician, and that this is all the more desirable when the great modern developments in technique tend to obscure the fundamental basis of clinical medicine. Not only was Hippocrates a great writer, a great teacher and a great observer, he was in the first place a great humanist. It is impossible to read these lectures and aphorisms without learning something of the greatness and charity of the art of medicine; there is still much here which is as valuable for the practice of medicine to-day as ever it was more than two thousand years ago in the islands of the Ægean Sea.

The plan of this book was first decided upon in 1941. The first attempts at translation were made auspiciously enough in

Alexandria, the scene of so much Hippocratic study; and although the collaborators continued to devote some of the leisure which war-time allowed to the task, only the peace of the last few years has made possible the final writing which is now at an end.

We wish to thank Miss P. M. Chasteney who prepared the manuscript for the press.

Oxford.   J. C.
London.   W. N. M.

CONTENTS

The Medical Works of Hippocrates

INTRODUCTION

HIPPOCRATES AND THE HIPPOCRATIC CORPUS

HIPPOCRATES is unquestionably a historic figure. He lived in the latter half of the fifth century B.C. in the Ægean island of Cos. Contemporary evidence shows that he was not only a famous physician, but taught medicine for fees. Further than that it is very difficult to go, for the scanty statements of Plato and of the anonymous author of a papyrus fragment are not definite enough to allow of more than speculation, while later evidence is unreliable.

Whatever the biographical facts which are lost, we have preserved a large collection of medical treatises which bear the name of Hippocrates and are known as the *Hippocratic Corpus*. The contents are very various: there are purely technical works, such as those on surgery; essays or lectures on various popular aspects of medicine, some polemic in tone; notes of actual cases; and a number of collections of short medical truths, of especial use in forecasting the course of an illness, which are exemplified by the *Aphorisms*. Here then is clearly not the work of one man, but a part at least of the library of an early Greek medical school, and tradition connects it with that of Cos. We must not be surprised therefore to find that the items vary much in style, content and value, including as they do some of the writings of a rival school at the neighbouring town of Cnidos. This collection or *corpus* seems to have been compiled and edited in the third or second centuries B.C. by the scholars of the famous library at Alexandria. Even so there is no single tradition; the order of the books is not the same in all our manuscripts and there is early evidence of

B

different arrangements. From that time on, critics have been fruitlessly engaged in trying to sort out the 'genuine' works of Hippocrates, and the authenticity of every one has been challenged at one time or another. This in itself is sufficient indication that the critics have no real criteria; and if the explanation of the *corpus* as the remains of a medical library is right, they are hardly likely to find any. None the less it is possible to sift the wheat from the chaff by the test of medical accuracy and worth, and all writers agree that some parts are the work of a great physician.

The vagaries of an Alexandrine editor may account for some apparent inconsistencies in the present volume. Thus we have translated only Books I and III of the seven entitled *Epidemics*, because it is generally agreed that these are the most valuable or 'genuine', and are probably by the same author, whereas the other books are not. It will also be apparent why almost all editions of Hippocrates are selections. The principles we have followed in presenting the present selection must be explained. In the first place we made the arbitrary rule of including only the medical works, thus omitting those parts which deal with surgery and obstetrics. Of the medical and general books we have chosen a representative selection of all that is best. We have omitted works which show, either by language or sense, that they are the products of a later age. We have also omitted some good works which are very similar to, or even largely repetitions of, works we have included. The choice, apart from the exclusion of the technical treatises on surgery and midwifery, is not so arbitrary as it would appear. The author of the *Science of Medicine*, or one of his school, could not have composed some of the obscure necromancy which is found among the books ascribed to Hippocrates.

HISTORICAL AND MEDICAL APPRECIATION

The name of Hippocrates has been associated with all that is best in the Western tradition of medicine ever since 400 B.C. His works were known and studied throughout the ancient world, even by men who were not professional physicians. Some acquaintance with the principles and even the practice of healing was expected in every educated man, an important accomplishment for the owner of a large establishment of slaves. Cato, it is true, with the characteristic brutal logic of the early Romans, recommended selling a slave who fell sick; but it was not long before an ingenious Greek thought of buying up sick slaves, treating them in his own hospital and selling them again when cured. Thus whatever the status of the physician (and Juvenal mentions him in the same breath with the acrobat and the astrologer), medicine enjoyed a high repute. Commentaries soon began to be written on the Hippocratic works, and those of Galen, dating from the second century A.D., still survive. Glossaries too were made of the medical terms, one of which compiled by Erotian in the time of Nero is also extant. But more than this, the pithy sayings of the *Aphorisms* were lifted from their context and generalized into proverbs: few now know that the well-known *ars longa, vita brevis* is a quotation from the *Aphorisms* (I, 1), and recollections of Hippocratic maxims may be recognized in the most unlikely places.

Greek medicine, for it remained predominantly Greek even under the Roman Empire, seems to have reached its zenith about the first century A.D. But it never advanced far in clinical practice beyond the Hippocratic stage, and it became in fact contaminated by charms and magical practices in the remedies to be found in the more popular books. Scientific detachment was the supreme contribution of Greece, and especially of Ionia, to the development of Western thought, and its expression in Hippocrates secured for him an enduring and well-earned fame. The fourth century A.D. saw a Latin version of some of the works; later on Syriac versions are known. Chaucer knew of 'Ypocras', and Dante includes him in his list of noted pagan scientists; Sir Thomas Browne, referring to the names and addresses in the *Epidemics*, asked: 'Who cares to subsist like Hippocrates' Patients . . . under naked nominations, without deserts or noble acts?'

As science emerged from the dark alchemy of the Middle Ages, the assimilation of Hippocratic notions into the *corpus* of modern medicine became an easy matter because the science we know to-day is the science of the Greeks; the facts more numerous, but the manner of their assessment the same. So it is difficult now to say of our present practice of clinical medicine that we owe this or that to Hippocrates, while some other methods belong to someone else. Rather did Hippocrates give a shape and direction to the practice of medicine, whether it was stating the ethical standards he demanded of the practitioner, or explaining in exact argument why epilepsy is a disease due to natural causes like any other, rather than a punishment inflicted by the gods. Nevertheless, it always comes as a surprise that many of our cherished clinical observations appear described with such clarity in the Hippocratic works. The reader will find for himself many examples, but the association of clubbed, or 'Hippocratic fingers' as they are sometimes called abroad, with suppuration within the chest; the significance of convulsions in infancy and the description of an epidemic of mumps are a few which come to mind. There are other passages which, though more obscure, in some ways have an even greater interest. Thus there is a suggestion that Hippocrates conceived of the experimental method as a means by which the secrets of nature might be discovered; in another passage, one might believe that he appreciated the phenomenon of allergy. In revising the translation, it was tempting, by a footnote or some other device, to call the attention of the reader to such passages. But it is easy to see something that perhaps is not there or to miss a truth that is concealed: we have left the reader to his own discoveries.

THE TEXT AND THE TRANSLATION

Books in Ancient Greece could only be made by individual copying. They were therefore not produced in any great numbers and there was always a chance of errors creeping in each time a new copy was made. As these faulty texts were themselves copied so the errors were multiplied and propagated; at the same time readers or copyists might make corrections either by conjecture or by comparison with another copy. Hippocrates has of course suffered much in this process which has preserved the works for us. Our earliest manuscript is probably of the tenth century A.D.; that is, it was written at least thirteen hundred years after the works it contains were composed. We have others of the eleventh and twelfth centuries and a number of less valuable later ones. From a comparison of these it is possible to reconstruct a fairly satisfactory text, but there will obviously be places where none of the manuscripts provides a likely reading or where they all fail. In the one case we must, if possible, restore by conjecture what was the probable text, in the other we can do nothing but signify the gap or *lacuna* by a row of asterisks. Some important chapters of *Airs, Waters and Places* are lost in this way. However, the researches of generations of scholars have succeeded in restoring what is on the whole a sound and reliable text. In translation we have done our best to avoid any discussion of dubious readings, selecting where possible that which seems to make the best sense. In one or two places we have varied the traditional order to improve the connection of thought. In a very few instances we have ventured to make new suggestions which we think are demanded by the sense; but in the main we have followed the best texts available. The text of Kuehlewein, in the Teubner series, Leipzig, 1895–1902, has been used for *Airs, Waters, Places, Ancient Medicine, Epidemics I* and *III* and *Regimen in Acute Diseases*. However, a number of works we wished to include are not given in this edition and for these we have relied upon the text of Dr. W. H. S. Jones, published in the Loeb Library (Volumes I, II and IV), London, 1923; for *Coan Prognosis*, upon that of Littré (Volume V), Paris, 1846.

The numbers of paragraphs and sections are traditional and have been inserted for the benefit of readers who wish to refer to the Greek texts or other translations.

The ideal translator of Hippocrates would have to be not only acquainted with Ancient Greek but also to have a wide knowledge of practical medicine. In these days such a combination must be extremely rare, and we hope we have found a satisfactory substitute in our close co-operation in the respective fields. The translation has gone through several stages. First a careful and literal rendering was made of the

Greek together with notes on the meaning and alternative interpretations; this was edited, taking careful note of the medical significance of the passage, and put into current English. This revision was then checked against the Greek original, and so on, until a mutually agreed form was reached. As far as possible we have used modern medical English, with the obvious limitations. In some cases the original Greek medical term is still in current use but it is no longer, as may be seen from the context, a correct translation, for in the course of time the word may have come to bear a more limited or even a changed meaning. Thus the Greek word *noma* means a gangrenous patch and in the Hippocratic text is used to describe this condition occurring on the tonsils. However, in current medical terminology the word is used exclusively to describe gangrene of the mouth or *cancrum oris*. It is clear that to use the English word 'noma' as a translation of the Greek word *noma* falsifies the sense. We have, however, avoided using the modern name of a disease where there is no evidence that Hippocrates appreciated its morbid identity. In such cases we have left the translation as literal as possible, and in one case we have kept the Greek word. Hippocrates refers frequently to a febrile malady he terms *causus*. It is certain that he included under this diagnosis a variety of fevers common in the Levant, but which we now separate into a number of different diseases. In many cases, enteric fever is clearly described; but as the condition, *causus*, cannot be generally identified as a single disease, the term is kept in the translation whenever it appears in the original text.

There are evident pitfalls in this joint method of translation. For instance, it is very easy, particularly in textually corrupt passages, to ascribe to Hippocrates an insight into morbid processes which he did not have. But we believe we have made few such mistakes. The alternative is to leave this selection and interpretation to the reader, but that was not our object in producing this new translation. The readers for whom this book is intended may not have the time nor opportunities to weigh and scrutinize each sentence; they will expect that to have been done for them, and they have here presented the best that the translators can provide. Nor need they fear that the necessary interpretation has obscured their view of the real Hippocrates; a glance at previous translations will show that this does not affect the major part of the work, or indeed the important conclusions.

A note on the system of counting days seems necessary. It was the Greek custom to include the days at both ends, so that the third day means the day after to-morrow, and so on—a meaning familiar in terms taken from Greek medicine such as tertian or quartan. It seems best, once this has been pointed out, to leave all the numbers as they appear in the Greek text; the reader must remember that the twentieth day, for example, means what we should in ordinary speech call the nineteenth.

In order to facilitate reference to Hippocrates to see what he said on specific topics we have taken particular pains with the index. To the ordinary index we have added a short index of diseases and conditions, to which, although not mentioned by name, it is evident or likely that passages in the text refer. Thus it will be possible for the student to look up in this index such subjects as *mumps* or *diphtheria* or the *inheritance of acquired characteristics* and find something about these subjects in the text. It must be realized that an index of this kind, depending on interpretation and sometimes reasonable guesswork, must be liable to a good deal of error; nevertheless it may add some interest for the modern student.

CHRONOLOGICAL NOTE

Hippocrates, writing 400 years before the introduction of the Julian calendar, had no convenient method for giving dates in the year. There were several different calendars in use in Greece, and they were all based upon lunar months, so that the same date would not always fall on the same day of the solar year. It was therefore common practice to use certain astronomical events as a rough method of dating. The four obvious points are the equinoxes and solstices: March 21, September 21, June 21, December 22. These are from time to time supplemented by reference to the heliacal rising or setting of certain stars and constellations. Owing to the precession of the equinoxes these are not constant, and various factors prevent an exact calculation of the dates Hippocrates intended. The chief of these mentioned in the text, together with their approximate equivalents, are:

The rising of Arcturus	–	September 10
The rising of the Pleiads	–	– May 10
The setting of the Pleiads	–	November 11
The rising of the Dog Star	–	– July 17

THE OATH

I SWEAR by Apollo the healer, by Æsculapius, by Health and all the powers of healing, and call to witness all the gods and goddesses that I may keep this Oath and Promise to the best of my ability and judgement.

I will pay the same respect to my master in the Science as to my parents and share my life with him and pay all my debts to him. I will regard his sons as my brothers and teach them the Science, if they desire to learn it, without fee or contract. I will hand on precepts, lectures and all other learning to my sons, to those of my master and to those pupils duly apprenticed and sworn, and to none other.

I will use my power to help the sick to the best of my ability and judgement; I will abstain from harming or wronging any man by it.

I will not give a fatal draught to anyone if I am asked, nor will I suggest any such thing. Neither will I give a woman means to procure an abortion.

I will be chaste and religious in my life and in my practice.

I will not cut, even for the stone, but I will leave such procedures to the practitioners of that craft.

Whenever I go into a house, I will go to help the sick and never with the intention of doing harm or injury. I will not abuse my position to indulge in sexual contacts with the bodies of women or of men, whether they be freemen or slaves.

Whatever I see or hear, professionally or privately, which ought not to be divulged, I will keep secret and tell no one.

If, therefore, I observe this Oath and do not violate it, may I prosper both in my life and in my profession earning good repute among all men for all time. If I transgress and forswear this Oath, may my lot be otherwise.

THE CANON

A brief note on the characteristics desirable in a student of medicine.

ALTHOUGH the art of healing is the most noble of all the arts, yet, because of the ignorance both of its professors and of their rash critics, it has at this time fallen into the least repute of them all. The chief cause for this seems to me to be that it is the only science for which states have laid down no penalties for malpractice. Ill-repute is the only punishment and this does little harm to the quacks who are compounded of nothing else. Such men resemble dumb characters on the stage who, bearing the dress and appearance of actors, yet are not so. It is the same with the physicians; there are many in name, few in fact.

For a man to be truly suited to the practice of medicine, he must be possessed of a natural disposition for it, the necessary instruction, favourable circumstances, education, industry and time. The first requisite is a natural disposition, for a reluctant student renders every effort vain. But instruction in the science is easy when the student follows a natural bent, so long as care is taken from childhood to keep him in circumstances favourable to learning and his early education has been suitable. Prolonged industry on the part of the student is necessary if instruction, firmly planted in his mind, is to bring forth good and luxuriant fruit.

The growth of plants forms an excellent parallel to the study of medicine. Our characters resemble the soil, our masters' precepts the seed; education is the sowing of the seed in season and the circumstances of teaching resemble the climatic conditions that control the growth of plants. Industrious toil and the passage of time strengthen the plant and bring it to maturity.

The man, then, who brings these qualities to the study of medicine and who has acquired an exact knowledge of the subject before he sets out to practise, must be considered a doctor not only in name but in fact. Want of skill is a poor thing to prize and treasure. It robs a man of contentment and tranquillity night and day and makes him prone to cowardice and recklessness, the one a mark of weakness, the other of ignorance. Science and opinion are two different things; science is the father of knowledge but opinion breeds ignorance.

Holy things are revealed only to holy men. Such things must not be made known to the profane until they are initiated into the mysteries of science.

TRADITION IN MEDICINE

*An explanation of the empirical basis of medicine as practised
about the end of the fifth century B.C.*

1. In all previous attempts to speak or to write about
medicine, the authors have introduced certain arbitrary sup-
positions into their arguments, and have reduced the causes
of death and the maladies that affect mankind to a narrow
compass. They have supposed that there are but one or two
causes; heat or cold, moisture, dryness or anything else they
may fancy. From many considerations their mistake is
obvious; indeed, this is proved from their own words. They
are specially to be censured since they are concerned with no
bogus science, but one which all employ in a matter of the
greatest importance, and one of which the good professors
and practitioners are held in high repute. But besides such
there are both sorry practitioners and those who hold widely
divergent opinions. This could not happen were medicine a
bogus science to which no consideration had ever been given
and in which no discoveries had been made. For if it were so,
all would be equally inexperienced and ignorant, and the
condition of their patients due to nothing but the law of
chance. But this is not so, and the practitioners of medicine
differ greatly among themselves both in theory and practice
just as happens in every other science. For this reason I do
not think that medicine is in need of some new hypothesis,
dealing, for instance, with invisible or problematic substances,
and about which one must have some theory or another in
order to discuss them seriously. In such matters, medicine
differs from subjects like astronomy and geology, of which
a man might know the truth and lecture on it without either
he or his audience being able to judge whether it were the
truth or not, because there is no sure criterion.

2. Medicine has for long possessed the qualities necessary
to make a science. These are original observations and a

known method according to which many valuable discoveries have been made over a long period of time. By such a method, too, the rest of the science will be discovered if anyone who is clever enough is versed in the observations of the past and makes these the starting point of his researches. If anyone should reject these and, casting them aside, endeavour to proceed by a new method and then assert that he has made a discovery, he has been and is being deceived. A discovery cannot be made thus, and the reason why such a thing is impossible I shall endeavour to show by expounding the true nature of the science. My exposition will demonstrate clearly the impossibility of making discoveries by any other method but the orthodox one.

It seems to me to be of the greatest importance that anyone speaking of the science should confine himself to matters known to the general public, since the subject of inquiry and discourse is none other than the maladies of which they themselves fall sick. Although it were no easy matter for common people to discover for themselves the nature of their own diseases and the causes why they get worse or get better, yet it is easy for them to follow when another makes the discoveries and explains the events to them. Then when a man hears about a disease he will only have to remember his own experience of it. But if anyone departs from what is popular knowledge and does not make himself intelligible to his audience, he is not being practical. For such reasons we have no need of hypotheses.

3. In the first place, the science of medicine would never have been discovered nor, indeed, sought for, were there no need for it. If sick men fared just as well eating and drinking and living exactly as healthy men do, and no better on some different regimen, there would be little need for the science. But the reason why the art of medicine became necessary was because sick men did not get well on the same regimen as the healthy, any more than they do now. What is more, I am of the opinion that our present way of living and our present diet would not have come about if it had proved adequate for a man to eat and drink the same things as an ox or a horse and

all the other animals. The produce of the earth, fruits, vegetables and grass, is the food of animals on which they grow and
flourish without needing other articles of diet. In the beginning I believe that man lived on such food and the modern
diet is the result of many years' discovery. Such devising was
necessary because, in primitive times, men often suffered
terribly from their indigestible and animal-like diet, eating raw
and uncooked food, difficult to digest. They suffered as men
would suffer now from such a diet, being liable to violent pain
and sickness and a speedy death. Certainly such ills would
probably prove less serious then than now because they were
accustomed to this kind of food, but even then, such illnesses
would have been serious and would have carried off the
majority of a weak constitution although the stronger would
survive longer, just as now some people easily digest strong
meats while others suffer much pain and illness from them.
For this reason I believe these primitive men sought food
suitable to their constitutions and discovered that which we
now use. Thus, they took wheat and wetted it, winnowed it,
ground it, sifted it, and then mixed it and baked it into bread,
and likewise made cakes from barley. They boiled and
baked and mixed and diluted the strong raw foods with the
weaker ones and subjected them to many other processes,
always with a view to man's nature and his capabilities. They
knew that if strong food was eaten the body could not digest
it and thus it would bring about pain, sickness and death,
whereas the body draws nourishment and thus grows and is
healthy from food it is able to digest. What fairer or more
fitting name can be given to such research and discovery than
that of medicine, which was founded for the health, preserva-
tion and nourishment of man and to rid him of that diet
which caused pain, sickness and death?

4. It is perhaps not unreasonable to assert that this is no
science, for no one can properly be called the practitioner of
a science of which the facts are unknown to none and with
which all are acquainted by necessity and experience. The
discoveries of medicine are of great importance and are the
result of thought and skill on the part of many people. For

instance, even now trainers in athletics continue to make discoveries according to the same method; they determine what men must eat and drink to gain the greatest mastery over their bodies and to achieve the maximum strength.

5. Turning now to what is generally admitted to be the science of medicine, namely, discoveries concerning the sick, which is a science in name and boasts practitioners, let us consider whether it has the same purposes and from what origins it arose. As I have already said, I do not believe anyone would ever have looked for such a science if the same regimen were equally good for the sick and the healthy. Even now some people, the barbarians and some Greeks, who have no knowledge of medicine, go on behaving when they are ill just as they do in health. They neither abstain from nor moderate the use of the things they like. Those who sought for and found the science of medicine held the same opinion as those whom I mentioned before. First of all, I imagine, they cut down the quantity without changing the quality of the food, making the sick eat very little. But when it became clear to them that such a regimen suited and helped some of the sick but not all, and that there were some even who were in such a condition that they could not digest even a very little food, then they concluded that in some cases a more easily digested food was necessary. Thus they invented gruel by mixing a little strong food with much water, so taking away its strength by dilution and cooking. For those that could not digest even gruel, they substituted liquid nourishment, taking care that this should be of moderate dilution and quantity, neither too weak nor too strong.

6. It must be clearly understood, however, that gruel is not necessarily of assistance to everyone who is sick. In some diseases it is evident that on such a diet, the fever and pains increase, the gruel serving as nourishment to the disease, but as a source of decline and sickness to the body. In such cases were dry food to be taken, barley-cakes or bread for example, even in very small quantities, the patients would become ten times worse than they would be on a diet of gruel, simply because of the strength of the food. Again, a man who was

helped by gruel but not by dry food would be worse if he ate none of the latter than if he took only a little, and even a small quantity would give him pain. In fact, it is obvious that all the causes of such pains come to the same thing; the stronger foods are the most harmful to man whether he be in health or sickness.

7. What then is the difference in intention between the man who discovered the mode of life suitable for the sick, who is called a physician and admitted to be a scientist, and him who, from the beginning, discovered the way to prepare the food we eat now instead of the former wild and animal-like diet? I can see no difference; the discovery is one and the same thing. The one sought to do away with those articles of diet which, on account of their savage and undiluted nature the human frame could not digest, and on which it could not remain healthy; the other discovered what a sick man could not digest in view of his particular malady. What difference is there save in the appearance, and that the one is more complicated and needs more study? Indeed, one is the fore-runner of the other.

8. A comparison between the diets of a sick man and a healthy one shows that the diet of a healthy man is no more harmful to a sick man than that of a wild beast to a healthy man. Suppose a man be suffering from a disease, neither something malignant nor incurable, nor yet some trifling ailment, but one nevertheless of which he is well aware. If he were to eat bread or meat or anything else which is nourishing to a healthy man, but in smaller quantities than if he were well, he would suffer pain and run some risk. Now suppose a healthy man were to take small quantities of a diet which would give strength and nourishment to an ox or a horse, such as vetch or barley-corn, he would suffer no less pain and run no less risk than the sick man who inopportunely ate bread or barley-cake. This proves that the whole science of medicine might be discovered by research according to these principles.

9. If it were all as simple as this, that the stronger foods are harmful and the weaker good and nourishing for men both in health and sickness, the matter were an easy one. The safest

course would be to keep to the weaker food. But if a man were to eat less than enough he would make as big a mistake as if he were to eat too much. Hunger is a powerful agent in the human body; it can maim, weaken and kill. Under-nourishment gives rise to many troubles and, though they are different from those produced by over-eating, they are none the less severe because they are more diverse and more specific. One aims at some criterion as to what constitutes a correct diet, but there is no standard by reference to which accuracy may be achieved; physical sensation is the only guide. Thus exactness is difficult to achieve and small errors are bound to occur. I warmly commend the physician who makes small mistakes; infallibility is rarely to be seen. Most doctors seem to me to be in the position of poor navigators. In calm weather they can conceal their mistakes, but when overtaken by a mighty storm or a violent gale, it is evident to all that it is their ignorance and error which is the ruin of the ship. So it is with the sorry doctors who are the great majority. They cure men but slightly ill, in whose treatment even the biggest mistakes would have no serious consequences. Such diseases are many and much more common than the more serious ones. When doctors make mistakes over such cases, their errors are unperceived by the layman, but when they have to treat a serious and dangerous case, a mistake or lack of skill is obvious to all, and vengeance for either error is not long delayed.

10. That over-eating should cause no less sickness than excessive fasting is easily understood by reference to the healthy. Some find it better to dine but once a day and consequently make this their custom. Others, likewise, find it is better for them to have a meal both at noon and in the evening. Then there are some who adopt one or other of these habits merely because it pleases them or because of chance circumstances. On the grounds of health it matters little to most people whether they take but one meal a day or two. But there are some who, if they do not follow their usual custom, do not escape the result and they may be stricken with a serious illness within a day. Some there are who, if they take luncheon when this practice does not agree with them,

C

at once become both mentally and physically dull; they yawn and become drowsy and thirsty. If subsequently they should dine as well, they suffer from wind, colic and diarrhoea and, not infrequently, this has been the start of a serious illness even though they have taken no more than twice the amount of food they have been accustomed to. Similarly, a man who is accustomed to taking luncheon because he finds that this agrees with him, cannot omit the meal without suffering great weakness, fear and faintness. In addition, his eyes become sunken, the urine more yellow and warmer, the mouth bitter, and he has a sinking feeling in his stomach. He feels dizzy, despondent and incapable of exertion. Then later when he sits down to dine, food is distasteful to him and he cannot eat his customary dinner. Instead, the food causes colic and rumblings and burns the stomach; he sleeps poorly and is disturbed by violent nightmares. With such people this too has often been the start of some illness.

11. Let us consider the reason for these things. The man who is accustomed to dine only once a day suffers, in my opinion, when he takes an extra meal because he has not waited long enough since the last. His stomach has not fully benefited from the food taken on the previous day and has neither digested nor discarded it, nor calmed down again. This new food is introduced into the stomach while it is still digesting and fermenting the previous meal. Such stomachs are slow in digestion and need rest and relaxation. The man who is accustomed to a meal at midday suffers when he has to go without, because his body needs nourishment and the food taken at the previous meal has already been used up. If no fresh food be taken his body wastes through starvation, and I attribute to this the symptoms from which I described such a man to suffer. I maintain that other healthy people will suffer from these same troubles if they fast for two or three days.

12. Those constitutions which react rapidly and severely to changes in habit are, in my opinion, the weak ones. A weak man is next to a sick man, while a sick man is made still weaker by indiscretions in his diet. In matters requiring such nicety, it is impossible for science to be infallible. There are many

things in medicine which require just as careful judgement as this matter of diet, and of these I will speak later. I contend that the science of medicine must not be rejected as non-existent or ill-investigated because it may sometimes fail in exactness. Even if it is not always accurate in every respect, the fact that it is able to approach close to a standard of infallibility as a result of reasoning, where before there was great ignorance, should command respect for the discoveries of medical science. Such discoveries are the product of good and true investigation, not chance happenings.

13. I wish now to return to those whose idea of research in the science is based upon a new method; the supposition of certain hypotheses. They would suppose that there is some principle harmful to man; heat or cold, wetness or dryness, and that the right way to bring about cures is to correct cold with warmth, or dryness with moisture and so on. On such an assumption let us consider the case of a man of weak constitution. Suppose he eats grains of wheat as they come straight from the threshing-floor and raw meat, and suppose he drinks water. If he continues with such a diet I am well aware that he will suffer terribly. He will suffer pain and his body will become enfeebled; his stomach will be disordered and he will not be able to live long. What remedy, then, should be employed for someone in this condition? Heat or cold or dryness or wetness? It must obviously be one of them because these are the causes of disease, and the remedy lies in the application of the opposite principle according to the hypothesis. Really, of course, the surest remedy is to stop such a diet and to give him bread instead of grains of wheat, cooked instead of raw meat and wine to drink with it. Such a change is bound to bring back health so long as this has not been completely wrecked by the prolonged consumption of his former diet. What conclusion shall we draw? That he was suffering from cold and the remedy cured him because it was hot, or the reverse of this? I think this is a question which would greatly puzzle anyone who asked it. What was taken away in preparing bread from wheat; heat, cold, moisture or dryness? Bread is subjected to fire and water and many other

things in the course of its preparation, each of which has its own effect. Some of the original qualities of wheat are lost, some are mixed and compounded with others.

14. I know too that the body is affected differently by bread according to the manner in which it is prepared. It differs according as it is made from pure flour or meal with bran, whether it is prepared from winnowed or unwinnowed wheat, whether it is mixed with much water or little, whether well mixed or poorly mixed, over-baked or under-baked, and countless other points besides. The same is true of the preparation of barley-meal. The influence of each process is considerable and each has a totally different effect from another. How can anyone who has not considered such matters and come to understand them, possibly know anything of the diseases that afflict mankind? Each one of the substances of a man's diet acts upon his body and changes it in some way and upon these changes his whole life depends, whether he be in health, in sickness, or convalescent. To be sure, there can be little knowledge more necessary. The early investigators in this subject carried out their researches well and along the right lines. They referred everything to the nature of the human body, and they thought such a science worthy of being ascribed to a god as is now believed. They never imagined that there was some 'principle' of heat or cold, of wetness or dryness, which either harmed a man or was necessary to his health. They attributed disease to some factor stronger and more powerful than the human body which the body could not master. It was such factors they sought to remove. Every quality is at its most powerful when it is most concentrated; sweetness at its sweetest, bitterness at its bitterest, sourness at its sourest and so forth. The existence of such qualities in the body of man was perceived together with their harmful effects. There exists in man saltness, bitterness, sweetness, sharpness, astringency, flabbiness and countless other qualities having every kind of influence, number and strength. When these are properly mixed and compounded with one another, they can neither be observed nor are they harmful. But when one is separated out and stands alone it becomes both apparent and

harmful. Similarly, the foods which are unsuitable for us and harm us if eaten, all have some such characteristic; either they are bitter or salt or sharp or have some other strong and undiluted quality. For that reason we are disturbed by them, just as similar qualities when retained in the body harm us. Those things which form the ordinary and usual food of man, bread and barley-cakes and the like, are clearly farthest removed from those things which have a strong or strange taste. In this way they differ from those that are prepared and designed for pleasure and luxury. The simple foods least often give rise to bodily disturbance and a separation of the forces located there. In fact, strength, growth and nourishment come from nothing but what is well mixed and contains no strong nor undiluted element.

15. I am utterly at a loss to know how those who prefer these hypothetical arguments and reduce the science to a simple matter of 'principles' ever cure anyone on the basis of their assumptions. I do not think that they have ever discovered anything that is purely 'hot' or 'cold', 'dry' or 'wet', without it sharing some other qualities. Rather, I fancy, the diets they prescribe are exactly the same as those we all employ, but they impute heat to one substance, cold to another, dryness to a third and wetness to a fourth. It would be useless to bid a sick man to 'take something hot'. He would immediately ask 'What?' Whereupon the doctor must either talk some technical gibberish or take refuge in some known solid substance. But suppose 'something hot' is also astringent, another is hot and soothing as well, while a third produces rumbling in the belly. There are many varied hot substances with many and varied effects which may be contrary one to another. Will it make any difference to take that which is hot and astringent rather than that which is hot and soothing, or even that which is cold and astringent or cold and soothing? To the best of my knowledge the opposite is the case; everything has its own specific effect. This is not only true of the human body but is seen in the various substances used for working hides and wood and other things less sensitive than flesh and blood. It is not the heating effect of the application which is so important

as its astringent or soothing qualities and so on, and this is true whether the substance be taken internally or applied as an ointment or plaster.

16. I think cold and heat are the weakest of the forces which operate in the body, and for these reasons. So long as cold and heat are present together they are harmless, for heat is tempered by cold and cold by heat. But when the two principles are separated from each other then they become harmful. However, when the body is chilled, warmth is spontaneously generated by the body itself so there is no need to take special measures, and this is true both in health and in disease. For instance, if a healthy man cools his body by taking a cold bath or any other means, the more he cools himself the warmer he feels when he resumes his garments and comes into shelter again. This is only true, of course, so long as he does not wholly freeze. Again if he should warm himself thoroughly with a hot bath or at a fire, and then go into a cool place, it will seem to be much colder than formerly and he will shiver more. Should anyone cool himself with a fan on a very hot day, the heat seems ten times more suffocating when the fan is stopped than if its cooling properties had not been used at all. Let us consider now a more extreme example. If people get their feet, hands or head frozen by walking through snow or from exposure to cold, think of what they suffer from burning and irritation at night when they are wrapped up and come into a warm place; in some cases blisters come up like those formed by a burn. But these things do not happen before they get warm. This shows how readily each of this pair replaces the other. There are countless other examples I might give to illustrate this subject. Is it not true of sick men that those who have the severest chill develop the highest fever? And even when the fever abates its fury a little, the patient remains very hot. Then subsequently as it passes through the body, it finishes in the feet, that is the first part of the body to be attacked by the chill and the part which remained cold the longest. Again when the patient sweats as the fever falls, he feels much colder than if he had not had the fever at all. What great or fearful effect, then, can a thing have when its opposite appears of itself

with such speed and removes any effect that the former may have had? What need is there, also, for further assistance when nature neutralizes the effect of such an agent spontaneously?

Some may raise the objection that the fever of patients suffering from *causus*, pneumonia or other serious diseases does not rapidly decline. Neither in such cases is the fever intermittent. I think that such observations constitute a good proof of my own view that a high temperature is not the only element of a fever nor the only cause of the weak constitution of a febrile patient. May it not be said of a thing that it is both bitter and hot, sharp and hot, salt and hot, and countless other combinations both with heat and cold. In each combination, the effect of any two qualities acting together will be different. Such qualities may be harmful but there is as well the heat of physical exertion which increases as the strength increases and has no ill effects.

18. The truth of this may be demonstrated by the following consideration of certain signs. An obvious one, and one we have all experienced and shall continue to do so, is that of the common cold. When we have a running at the nose and there is a discharge from the nostrils, the mucus is more acrid than that which is present when we are well. It makes the nose swell and renders it hot and inflamed. The fever does not fall when the nose is running, but when the discharge becomes thicker, less acrid, milder and more of its ordinary consistency. Similar changes may be seen as the result of cold alone, but the same observations can be made. There is the same change from cold to hot and hot to cold and the changes take place readily. I assert too that all other illnesses that are caused by acrid or undiluted humours within the body follow a similar course; they subside as these humours become less potent and are diluted.

19. Those humours which affect the eyes are very acrid and cause sores upon the eyelids; sometimes they cause destruction of the cheeks and the parts beneath the eyes. The discharge destroys anything it may touch even eating away the clothes around the face. Pain, heat and swelling obtain until such time

as the discharges are 'digested' and become thicker and give rise to a serum. The process of 'digestion' is due to their being mixed and diluted with one another and warmed together. Again, the humours of the throat which cause hoarseness and sore throats, those of erysipelas or pneumonia are at first salt, moist and acrid and during this phase the maladies flourish. But when the discharges become thicker and milder and lose their acridity, the fevers cease as well as the other effects of the disease which are harmful to the body. The cause of these maladies is found in the presence of certain substances, which, when present, invariably produce such results. But when the nature of these substances becomes changed, the illness is at an end. Any abnormal condition which arose purely as a result of heat or cold and into which no other factor entered at all would be resolved when a change occurred from hot to cold or *vice versa*. However, the changes which take place really occur in the manner I described above. All the ills from which man suffers are due to the operation of 'forces'. For instance, if a sufferer from biliousness, complaining of nausea, fever and weakness, gets rid of a certain bitter material which we call yellow bile either by himself or with the assistance of purging, it is evident how he gets rid of both the fever and the pain at the same time. As long as this material is un-absorbed and undiluted, no device will terminate either the pain or the fever. When there are pungent rust-coloured acids present in the body, there is frenzy and severe pain in the bowels and in the chest which cannot be cured until they have been purged of the acrid humours responsible and their poisonous effects neutralized by being mixed with other fluids. It is in the processes of digestion, change, dilution or thicken-ing by which the nature of a humour is altered that the causes of disease lie. It is for this reason that the occurrence of crises and the periodicity of certain diseases are so important. It is most improper that all these changes should be attributed to the effects of heat and cold, for such principles are not subject to degeneration or thickening. The changes of disease cannot be due to the effect of varying mixtures of such principles, for the only thing that will mix with heat and reduce its warmth

is coldness and *vice versa*. The various forces in the body
become milder and more health-giving when they are adjusted
to one another. A man is healthiest when these factors are
co-ordinated and no particular force predominates.

20. I think I have discussed this subject sufficiently, but
there are some sophists and learned men who maintain that
no one can understand the science of medicine unless he
knows what man is; that anyone who proposes to treat men
for their illnesses must first learn of such things. Their discourse then tends to philosophy as may be seen in the writings
of Empedocles and all the others who have ever written about
Nature; they discuss the origins of man and of what he was
created. It is my opinion that all which has been written by
doctors or sophists on Nature has more to do with painting
than medicine. I do not believe that any clear knowledge of
Nature can be obtained from any source other than a study of
medicine and then only through a thorough mastery of this
science. It is my intention to discuss what man is and how he
exists because it seems to me indispensable for a doctor to have
made such studies and to be fully acquainted with Nature. He
will then understand how the body functions with regard to
what is eaten and drunk and what will be the effect of any
given measure on any particular organ. It is not enough to
say 'cheese is harmful because it produces pain if much of it
is eaten'. One should know what sort of pain, why it is
produced and which organ of the body is upset. There are
many other harmful items of food and drink which affect the
body in different ways. For example, the taking of large
quantities of undiluted wine has a certain effect upon the body
and it is recognized, by those who understand, that the wine is
the cause and we know which organs are particularly affected.
I want to show that the same sort of thing is true of other
cases. Cheese, since that is the example I used, is not equally
harmful to all. Some can eat their fill of it without any unpleasant consequences and those whom it suits are wonderfully
strengthened by it. On the other hand, there are some who
have difficulty in digesting it. There must, then, be a difference
in their constitutions and the difference lies in the fact that,

in the latter case, they have something in the body which is inimical to cheese and this is aroused and disturbed by it. Those who have most of this humour and in whom it is at its strongest, naturally suffer most. If cheese were bad for the human constitution in general, it would affect everyone.

21. Both during convalescence as well as in the course of prolonged illnesses, complications are often seen. Some of them occur naturally in the course of the disease, others are occasioned by some chance happening. Most doctors, like laymen, tend to ascribe some such event to some particular activity that has been indulged in. In the same way they may ascribe something as being due to an alteration in their habits of bathing or walking or a change of diet, whether this is the actual case or not. As a result of jumping to conclusions, the truth may escape them. One must know with exactitude what is the effect of a bath or of fatigue indulged in at the wrong time. Neither such actions, nor eating too much, nor eating the wrong food will always produce the same effects; it depends upon other factors as well. No one who is unacquainted with the specific effects of such action on the body in different circumstances can know the results which follow and consequently cannot make proper use of them as therapeutic measures.

22. I think it should also be known what illnesses are due to 'forces' and what to 'forms'. By 'forces' I mean those changes in the constitution of the humours which affect the working of the body; by 'forms' I mean the organs of the body. Some of the latter are hollow and show variations in diameter, being narrow at one end and wide at the other, some are elongated, some solid and round, some flat and suspended, some are stretched out, some large, some thick, some are porous and sponge-like. For instance, which type of hollow organ should be the better able to attract and absorb moisture from the rest of the body: those which are all broad or those which are wide in part and narrow down? The latter kind. Such things have to be deduced from a consideration of external appearances and from anatomy. For instance, if you gape with your mouth wide open you cannot suck up any

fluid, but if you pout and compress the lips and then insert a
tube you can easily suck up as much as you like. Again,
cupping glasses are made concave for the purpose of drawing
and pulling the flesh up within them, and there are other examples
of this kind of thing. Among the inner organs of the body,
the bladder, the skull and the womb have such a shape and it
is well known that these organs specially attract moisture from
other parts of the body and are always filled with fluid. On
the other hand organs which are more spread out, although
they hold fluid which flows into them well, do not attract it to
the same extent. Further, the solid and round organs neither
attract it nor hold it because there is nowhere for the fluid to
lodge. Those which are spongy and of loose texture such as
the spleen, the lungs and the female breasts easily absorb
fluid from the nearby parts of the body and when they do so
become hard and swollen. Such organs do not absorb fluid and
then discharge it day after day as would a hollow organ containing fluid, but when they have absorbed fluid and all the
spaces and interstices are filled up, they become hard and tense
instead of soft and pliant. They neither digest the fluid nor
discharge it, and this is the natural result of their anatomical
construction. The organs of the body that cause flatulence and
colic, such as the stomach and chest, produce noise and
rumbling. For any hollow organ that does not become full of
fluid and remain so but instead undergoes changes and movement, must necessarily produce noises and the signs of movement. The organs which are soft and fleshy tend to become
obstructed and then they are liable to sluggishness and fullness.
Sometimes an organ which is diseased comes up against some
flat tissue which is neither strong enough to resist the force
of the swollen organ nor sufficiently mobile to accommodate
the diseased organ by yielding. For instance, the liver is tender,
full-blooded and solid and on account of these qualities is
resistant to the movement of other organs. Thus wind, being
obstructed by it, becomes more forceful and attacks the thing
which obstructs it with greater power. In the case of an organ
such as the liver, which is both full-blooded and tender, it
cannot but experience pain. For this reason, pain in the hepatic

area is both exceedingly severe and frequently encountered. Abscesses and tumours also occur very commonly here, as well as beneath the diaphragm. This latter condition, although less common, is more serious. The extent of the diaphragm is considerable and is opposed to other organs; nevertheless, its more sinewy and stronger nature makes it less liable to pain although both pains and tumours may occur in this region.

23. There are many individual variations in the shape of the different organs of the body from one person to another and they react differently both in health and in disease. There are large and small heads; thin and thick, long and short necks. The belly may be large and round; the chest narrow and flat. There are countless other differences and the effects of such variation must be known so that one can understand the exact cause when they become diseased. Only thus can proper care be given.

24. Again, the effect of each type of humour on the body must be learnt and, as I said before, their relationships with one another must be understood. I mean this sort of thing: if a sweet humour should change its nature, not by admixture with something else but spontaneously, what characteristic would it show? Bitter, salt, astringent or sharp? Sharp, I fancy. A sharp humour, compared with the others, would be specially inimical to the digestion of food. At least it would be so if, as we believe, a sweet humour is the most suited.

Thus, if anyone were able to light upon the truth by experiment outside the body, he would always be able to make the best pronouncements of all. The best advice is that which is least unsuitable.

EPIDEMICS, BOOK I

The Hippocratic Corpus *contains seven books of a physician's case notes. They consist of descriptions of both individual cases and diseases epidemic in a specified place in a given period. Books I and III appear to be the earliest and most interesting, and date from the fifth century B.C.; the other five books are probably the work of at least two later authors.*

(i)

1. There was much rain in Thasos about the time of the autumnal equinox and during the season of the Pleiads. It fell gently and continuously and the wind was from the South. During the winter, the wind blew mostly from the South; winds from the North were few and the weather was dry. On the whole the winter was like springtime; but the spring was cold with southerly[1] winds and there was little rain. The summer was for the most part cloudy but there was no rain. The etesian winds were few and light and blew at scattered intervals.[2]

Although the climate was generally southerly and dry, in the early spring there was a northerly spell, the very opposite of the previous weather. During this time a few people contracted *causus* without being much upset by it, and a few had haemorrhages but did not die of them. Many people suffered from swellings near the ears, in some cases on one side only, in others both sides were involved. Usually there was no fever and the patient was not confined to bed. In a few cases there was slight fever. In all cases the swellings subsided without harm and none suppurated as do swellings caused by other disorders. The swellings were soft, large and spread widely; they were unaccompanied by inflammation or pain and they disappeared leaving no trace. Boys, young men and male adults in the prime of life were chiefly affected and of these,

---

[1] Possibly a copyist's error for 'northerly'.
[2] The etesian winds blow from the north-west for forty days in the summer.

those given to wrestling and gymnastics were specially liable. Few women took it. Many patients had dry, unproductive coughs and hoarse voices. Soon after the onset of the disease, but sometimes after an interval, one or both testicles became inflamed and painful. Some had fever, but not all. These cases were serious enough to warrant attention, but for the rest, there were no illnesses requiring care.

2. During the period beginning in early summer and lasting into the winter, many patients with long-standing consumption took to their beds, for in many cases in which the diagnosis had been dubious, it was then confirmed. Some who had a consumptive diathesis, first began to suffer from the disease at that time. Many died including most of the latter, and of those who took to their beds I doubt if any survived even a moderate time. Death occurred more quickly than is usual in such cases. Other diseases, even the longer ones and those accompanied by fever, proved neither serious nor fatal; these will be described later. Only consumption was widespread and caused a large number of deaths.

In the majority of cases the course of the disease was as follows. There was fever, attended by shivering, of continuous, severe and usually non-remittent type. However the fever showed some variation of tertian periodicity. Thus one day the fever would be less severe, the next day the fever would be higher and so on, but in general becoming worse with time. The patients showed continuous sweating but the whole of the body was not involved. The extremities were often cold and could be warmed only with difficulty. Their stomachs were disordered and the stools small, bilious, not homogeneous, fluid and pungent, causing the patient to get up frequently. The urine was either thin, colourless and undigested, or thick with a slight sediment which did not settle easily but was, as it were, raw and unripe. Cough was slight but frequent, and little was coughed up and that only with difficulty. In the most violent cases, there was no progress towards ripening of the sputum and the patients continued to cough it up raw. In most of these cases the throat was painful, red and inflamed from the first and continued so. The stools were small, thin and pungent. The patients rapidly became worse and wasted away, refusing to take food and having no thirst. Many became delirious shortly before death.

3. While it was still summer and during the autumn there were also many cases of fever apart from consumption. These were continuous but not violent and, though those affected were ill for a long time, they suffered nothing in other respects for their stomachs generally remained in good order and they took no harm worth speaking of. Usually the urine was clear and of a good colour but thin, becoming ripened later about the time of the crisis. There was not too much coughing, nor did the patients have much trouble with the cough. They retained their appetites and it was quite permissible to give them food. Generally they were only slightly ill and showed none of the fevers attended with shivering suffered by consumptive patients, and little sweating. The paroxysms of fever were irregular, being at different intervals in different cases. In the shortest illnesses, the crisis occurred at about the twentieth day, in most cases at about the fortieth and in a number at about the eightieth. In some cases the fever resolved at a time different from those given above without reaching a crisis. In most of these the fever returned after a short interval and the crisis was reached in one of the usual periods. In many cases the malady was so protracted that it lasted into the winter.

Of all the diseases described in this section, only consumption proved fatal. The course of the remainder was smooth and no deaths occurred from the other fevers.

(ii)

4. There was unseasonably wintry weather in Thasos early in the autumn, and rainstorms suddenly burst to the accompaniment of northerly and southerly winds. This happened during the season of the Pleiads until their setting. The winter was northerly and there was much rain, with frequent heavy showers, as well as snow. Usually there were bright intervals as well, and the cold weather could not be regarded as unseasonable. However, immediately after the winter solstice

when the west wind usually begins to blow, the great storms
returned with gales from the north, and snow and rain fell
continuously from a sky full of racing clouds. This continued
without a break until the equinox. The spring was cold with
northerly winds accompanied by cloudy skies and much rain.
The summer was not too scorching for the etesian winds blew
steadily, but heavy rain followed again soon after the rising of
Arcturus.

5. The whole year then was wet, cold and northerly. The
winter was healthy for the most part but early in the spring
a good few, in fact most people, fell sick. Ophthalmia was the
first disease to make its appearance, being accompanied by
pain, moist discharge and without suppuration. Many people
had small styes break out which gave them trouble. Most
relapsed but were finally cured late in the year towards autumn.
During the summer and the autumn there were cases of
dysentery, tenesmus and diarrhoea. Further there were cases
of bilious diarrhoea in which the stools were copious, thin,
raw and sometimes watery and painful to pass. There were
also many cases of perineal abscess accompanied by strangury
and a painful, bilious, watery discharge containing particles
and pus. There was no disease of the kidneys (in these cases.)
Cases were seen in which there was vomiting of phlegm, bile
and undigested food. Sweating occurred and the patients
became flaccid all over. Often there was no fever and the
patients were not confined to bed, but in many other cases
which will be described there was fever. Those who exhibited
all the symptoms to be mentioned were consumptive and
suffered pain. During the autumn and on into the winter there
were cases of continued fever, in a few cases *causus*, diurnal
and nocturnal fevers, roughly tertian and exact tertian fevers,
quartans and fevers of no regular form. There were many
cases of each of the fevers about to be described.

6. *Causus* was the least frequent of these fevers and those
affected by it suffered the least. There was no bleeding, except
in a very few cases and then only very slight; nor was there
any delirium and in other respects all went well. The crisis
was regularly attained, usually on the seventeenth day including

the days of intermission. I knew of no case of *causus* which was fatal or which was complicated by brain-fever.

The tertian fevers were more common than *causus* and more troublesome. In all cases of this fever four periods regularly elapsed from the time the malady was contracted and the final crisis was reached after seven paroxysms. None suffered from relapses.

The quartan fevers showed, in many cases, their quartan nature from the start. In not a few cases, however, they emerged as quartans only on the departure of other fevers and ailments. As is usual they were long protracted, perhaps even more than usual.

There were many cases of quotidian, nocturnal and irregular fever; they lasted a long time whether the patients were confined to bed or not. In most cases the fever lasted through the season of the Pleiads until the winter. Often the disease was accompanied by convulsions, especially in the case of children when the fever was, at first, slight. Convulsions also sometimes followed the fever. Although these maladies were protracted, they were not usually serious unless the patient was already likely to die from some other cause.

7. The worst, most protracted and most painful of all the diseases then occurring were the continued fevers. These showed no real intermissions although they did show paroxysms in the fashion of tertian fevers, one day remitting slightly and becoming worse the next. They began mildly but continually increased, each paroxysm carrying the disease a stage further. A slight remission would be followed by a worse paroxysm and the malady generally became worse on the critical days. Although all patients suffering from these various fevers showed shivering fits at irregular times, such fits were least frequent and most irregular in patients with these continued fevers. Again, the fevers generally were attended with many fits of sweating but in cases of continued fever they were infrequent and brought harm rather than relief. In continued fever, too, the extremities were chilled and could only be warmed with difficulty, and insomnia was followed by coma. In the fevers generally, digestion was disturbed and

D

difficult but this was most marked in these cases of continued fever. In them, too, the urine was either: (*a*) Thin, raw and colourless becoming slightly more concocted at a crisis, (*b*) thick, but cloudy rather than forming sediment, or (*c*) of small quantity, bad and forming a raw sediment. Urine of this last variety was the most serious. Cough accompanied the fever, but I have no instance to record of a cough being either harmful or helpful.

8. These various symptoms (in cases of continued fever) were usually long-lasting, distressing and occurred without any order or regularity. In the majority of cases there was no crisis, whether or not the case was desperate. Some showed a brief respite but a relapse quickly followed. In a few cases a crisis occurred not earlier than the eightieth day but in some of these there was a relapse so that the majority of cases lasted on into the winter. Generally the disease resolved without a crisis, and this absence of crisis was equally marked both in those who recovered and those who did not.

These cases of (continued) fever, although they showed this characteristic of not reaching a crisis, were otherwise very varied. The most important and most ominous sign, which in the end was seen in most cases, was complete loss of appetite. This was specially marked in those whose condition was already desperate in other respects. Further, these febrile patients showed no greater desire for water than they would normally. Abscesses formed in those cases in which the illness was very prolonged and attended by much pain and loss of weight. These were so large, in some cases, as to be insufferable, while others were too small to be any good so that the patient soon returned to his former condition and deterioration was hastened.

9. This disease was commonly complicated by dysentery, tenesmus and diarrhoea. Some patients showed dropsy with or without these other symptoms. A violent attack of any of these complications quickly proved fatal; less severe attacks did no good. The disease was sometimes accompanied by transient eruptions, quite out of keeping with scale of the disease, and by swellings near the ears which slowly absorbed

and signified nothing. In some cases similar swellings occurred in the joints, especially the hips. Usually in such cases a crisis was reached in a few days and the swelling disappeared, only to regain a hold and quickly return to the original state.

10. All the diseases described caused death, but the greater number was among those suffering from this continued fever and especially children, including infants, older children and those approaching puberty. The complications described latterly were invariably accompanied by the general symptoms of the disease as at first described. On the other hand, many who suffered from these symptoms did not suffer the complications. The most important sign, and the only good one, which saved many who were in the gravest danger, was when strangury occurred and a local abscess was produced. Strangury, in these conditions, occurred most commonly at the ages mentioned above but in many other cases as well, both when the patient was confined to bed and when he was not. In those who showed this symptom, a rapid and violent change took place, for the belly, even though it might have been malignantly moist, rapidly became firm, while the patient's appetite for all kinds of food fully returned and the fever thereafter was mild. But even in these cases, the strangury lasted long and was painful, the urine being copious, thick, varied, red, mixed with pus and passed with pain. Nevertheless, all these patients recovered; I do not know of one who died.

11. Whenever there is danger, watch out for all ripe discharges that flow from every part of the body at their due times and for favourable and critical abscess formation. Ripeness shows that the crisis is at hand and that recovery is certain. On the other hand, what is raw and immature, as well as unfavourable abscess formation, denotes the failure to reach a crisis, pain, prolongation of the malady, death or relapse. To decide which course is likely you must consider other things too. Consider what has gone before, recognize the signs before your eyes and then make your prognosis. Study these principles. Practise two things in your dealings with disease: either help or do not harm the patient. There are

three factors in the practice of medicine: the disease, the patient and the physician. The physician is the servant of the science, and the patient must do what he can to fight the disease with the assistance of the physician.

12. Headache and pains in the neck, and a feeling of heaviness accompanied by pain, may occur both in the presence and in the absence of fever. Those suffering from brain fever have convulsions and vomit brownish-red material and some of these die rapidly. If a patient has a pain in the neck, heaviness in the temples, dimness of vision and contraction of the hypochondrium without pain, he will have an epistaxis, both in *causus* and in other fevers. If his whole head is heavy or he feels heartburn and nausea, he will vomit bilious and mucoid matter. In these diseases, convulsions are more common among children, both convulsions and uterine pain occur in women, while older patients and all whose warmth is disappearing suffer from paralysis, madness or loss of sight.

(iii)

13. A little before the rising of Arcturus and during its season there were many violent rainstorms in Thasos accompanied by northerly winds. About the time of the equinox and until the setting of the Pleiads, the winds were southerly, so little rain fell. The winter was northerly with periods of drought, cold, high winds and snow. There were very severe storms at the time of the equinox. The spring was northerly, dry, with little rain, and it was cold. There was little rain at the time of the summer solstice but instead a severe cold spell set in and lasted till the (rising of the) Dog Star. Thence, until the (rising of) Arcturus, the summer was hot. This hot spell began suddenly and was both continuous and severe. There was no rain and the etesian winds blew. About the time of Arcturus, southerly rains began and continued until the equinox.

14. Under such circumstances, cases of paralysis started to appear during the winter and became common constituting an epidemic. Some cases were swiftly fatal. In other respects, health remained good. Cases of *causus* were encountered early

in the spring and continued past the equinox towards summer. Most of those who fell sick in the spring or at the very beginning of summer recovered, though a few died. In the autumn, when the rains came, the disease was more fatal and the majority of those that took it died.

It is a peculiarity of *causus* that a good copious epistaxis often proved a cure, and I do not know of any in these circumstances who died if they had a good epistaxis. For Philiscus, Epameinon and Silenus had a small epistaxis on the fourth and fifth days; they died. Most of those who were sick had shivering attacks about the time of the crisis, especially those who did not have epistaxis. Such patients also had attacks of sweating.

15. Some cases of *causus* developed jaundice on the sixth day and these were assisted by diuresis, abdominal disturbance or by a profuse haemorrhage, such as Heracleides (who lay at Aristocydes' house) had. Moreover in this case he did not only have epistaxis but trouble in the belly and diuresis as well. He reached a crisis on the twentieth day. The servant of Phanagoras was not so lucky; he had none of these things happen to him and he died.

Most patients suffered from haemorrhage and especially was this the case in youths and young men. Indeed, of the latter who did not have a haemorrhage, most died. In older people the disease turned to jaundice or their bellies were upset, as was the case of Bion, who lay at Silenus' house. During the summer, dysentery became epidemic and those who had not recovered by that time had their sickness end up as a sort of dysentery, even when they had had a haemorrhage. This happened to Myllus and to Erato's slave whose illness, after a copious haemorrhage, turned to a sort of dysentery; they survived.

In fact, in this disease, this fluid was peculiarly abundant. Even those who did not bleed about the time of the crisis suffered pain and passed thin urine at this time and then began to bleed slightly about the twenty-fourth day, and there was pus mixed with the blood. In the case of Antiphon the son of Critobulus this finally ceased and the ultimate crisis was reached about the fortieth day. Such cases showed hard swellings near the ears which absorbed and were followed by a heaviness in the left flank and in the region of the iliac crest.

16. Many women were sick, but fewer women than men, and the disease in them was less fatal. Child-birth was often difficult and was followed by disease. These cases were specially fatal as, for instance, in that of the daughter of Telebulus, who died on the sixth day after giving birth. In most cases menorrhagia occurred during the fever and in many girls in whom menstruation was not previously established, but some had epistaxis. In some cases both menorrhagia and epistaxis were observed. For instance, the daughter of Daitharses who was a virgin not only had uterine bleeding for the first time then but also had a violent discharge of blood from the nose. I know of no case which proved fatal if either of these complications ensued. So far as I know, all who fell ill while pregnant aborted.

17. Generally in this disease the urine was of good colour but thin with a slight sediment. The belly was disordered, the stools being thin and bilious. In many cases, after a crisis had been reached for other disorders, the malady ended up as dysentery, as happened to Xenophanes and Critias. I will record the names of those patients who had watery, copious and fine urine, even after the crisis, with a healthy sediment, and who had a favourable crisis in other respects too. They were Bion, who lay at the home of Silenus; Cratis, who was at the house of Xenophanes; the slave of Areto, and the wife of Mnesistratus. All these subsequently suffered from dysentery.

About the time of Arcturus many reached the crisis on the eleventh day and they did not suffer the expected relapses. About this time, especially in children, the malady was associated with coma and these cases were the most rarely fatal of all.

18. *Causus* lasted on to the equinox, up to the setting of the Pleiads, and even into the winter. But at this time brain fever became prevalent and most of its victims died. A few similar cases were also seen during the summer. Those suffering from fever of the *causus* type which proved fatal showed certain

additional symptoms even at the beginning of the illness. High fever attended the beginning of the illness along with slight shivering fits, insomnia, thirst, nausea and a little sweating about the forehead and over the clavicles (in no case all over), much delirium, fears and despondency, while the extremities such as the toes were chilled, but especially the hands. Paroxysms occurred on even days. Generally, pain was greatest on the fourth day and the sweat was cold. Their extremities did not regain warmth but remained cold and livid, and they no longer suffered from thirst. They passed little urine, which was black and fine, and became constipated. In none of these cases was there a discharge of blood from the nose but only a few drops. Nor did these cases show any remission but died on the sixth day, sweating. Those patients who developed brain fever had all the above symptoms, but the crisis usually took place on the eleventh day. Where brain fever was not present at the beginning but appeared on the third or fourth day, the crisis did not take place until the twentieth day. In these the illness was moderate in its severity at first but became severe about the seventh day.

19. The disease was very widespread. Of those who contracted it death was most common among youths, young men, men in the prime of life, those with smooth skins, those of a pallid complexion, those with straight hair, those with black hair, those with black eyes, those who had been given to violent and loose living, those with thin voices, those with rough voices, those with lisps and the choleric. Many women also succumbed to this malady. During this epidemic there were four signs which betokened recovery; a considerable epistaxis, a large diuresis in which the urine contained a lot of favourable sediment, biliousness and disorders of the belly coming on at a favourable time, or if there were dysentery. In many cases the crisis was not reached upon the appearance of one of the symptoms described, but instead the symptoms appeared successively and the patients seemed to be in a very bad way. But in every such case they recovered. All these symptoms were seen in women and girls and if either any of them appeared or there was copious uterine haemorrhage, it

proved their salvation and brought on the crisis. I do not know of any woman who died in which one of these signs had properly appeared. However, the daughter of Philo had a severe epistaxis, but she dined rather intemperately on the seventh day of her sickness; she died.

If a patient weeps in spite of himself in acute fevers of the type of *causus*, you must expect an epistaxis, even if there is no other reason to expect a fatal outcome. If a patient be poorly, it portends not haemorrhage but death.

20. Swelling near the ears which sometimes accompanied fevers did not always subside or suppurate when the fever was resolved by crisis, but subsided following bilious diarrhoea or dysentery or by the formation of sediment in the urine as happened in the case of Hermippus of Clazomenae. The times of the crises in these fevers, which is the thing by which we distinguish them, were sometimes an even and sometimes an odd number of days. Thus, two brothers who lay near the summer residence of Epigenes fell sick at the same time. The elder reached a crisis on the sixth day, the younger on the seventh. Both relapsed at the same time following an intermission of five days. After the relapse they reached a crisis together on the seventeenth day from the beginning of the illness. Generally the crisis was attained on the sixth day and, following an intermission of six days, a second crisis was reached on the fifth day of the relapse. In some cases the crisis took place on the seventh day, the intermission lasted seven days and the relapse reached its crisis in three days. In others, the crisis occurred on the seventh day, and a second on the seventh day of the relapse which followed three days' intermission of fever. In some cases a crisis took place on the sixth day, the remission lasted six days and this was followed by three days' relapse, a remission of one day, a relapse of one day and finally the crisis. This happened to Evagon, the son of Daitharses. In other cases, a crisis took place on the sixth day, the remission lasted seven days with crisis on the fourth day of the relapse, as happened to the daughter of Aglaïdas. The majority of those who caught this epidemic passed their illness in the manner described and I know of none that survived

who did not have a relapse in the normal way. All who had relapses of this sort recovered so far as I know. Further, to my knowledge, none whose malady proceeded in this manner subsequently suffered a return of the disease.

21. In these fevers, death usually took place on the sixth day, as happened in the case of Epaminondas, Silenus and Philiscus the son of Antagoras. Those who had a swelling near the ears had a crisis on the twentieth day but in all cases it subsided without suppuration, being voided in the urine. Cratistonax, who lived near the temple of Heracles, and the servant girl of Scymnus the fuller developed abscesses; they died. In some cases the crisis was on the seventh day, and following nine days' remission the fever recurred and reached its crisis on the fourth day after the recurrence; this happened in the case of Pantacles who lived near the temple of Dionysus. Sometimes the first crisis was on the seventh day, the remission lasted six days and a crisis was reached on the seventh day of the recrudescence; this happened in the case of Phanocritus who lay at the home of Gnathon the fuller.

22. During the winter, from about the time of the winter solstice till the equinox, *causus* and brain fever continued, and there were many deaths. There was, however, a change in the periods at which the crisis occurred, it taking place usually on the fifth day from the beginning of the illness. A remission of four days would be followed by a relapse with the crisis on the fifth day, that is on the fourteenth day of the illness. Most of those who behaved in this way were children, but it happened occasionally in adults. In some cases a crisis occurred on the eleventh day, a relapse on the fourteenth and the final crisis on the twentieth. But if shivering fits supervened about the twentieth day, the crisis took place on the fortieth. Most patients suffered from shivering fits about the time of the first crisis, and those who had them then also had them at the time of the crisis of the relapse. Very few had shivering fits during the spring, more had them during the summer, still more during the autumn but by far the greatest number during the winter. Cases of haemorrhage gradually ceased.

23. The factors which enable us to distinguish between diseases are as follows: First we must consider the nature of man in general and of each individual and the characteristics of each disease. Then we must consider the patient, what food is given to him and who gives it—for this may make it easier for him to take or more difficult—the conditions of climate and locality both in general and in particular, the patient's customs, mode of life, pursuits and age. Then we must consider his speech, his mannerisms, his silences, his thoughts, his habits of sleep or wakefulness and his dreams, their nature and time. Next, we must note whether he plucks his hair, scratches or weeps. We must observe his paroxysms, his stools, urine, sputum and vomit. We look for any change in the state of the malady, how often such changes occur and their nature, and the particular changes which induce death or a crisis. Observe, too, sweating, shivering, chill, cough, sneezing, hiccough, the kind of breathing, belching, wind, whether silent or noisy, haemorrhages and haemorrhoids. We must determine the significance of all these signs.

24. Some fevers are continuous, others come at day and remit at night; others for the night, remitting by day. There are sub-tertian, tertian and quartan fevers, five-day, seven-day and nine-day fevers. The most severe, serious, troublesome and fatal maladies produce continued fevers. The safest, easiest to bear and yet longest of all is the quartan fever, not only from its own nature but also because it puts an end to other serious illnesses. What is termed sub-tertian fever can occur in acute illnesses, and it is the most fatal of all; but consumption and other protracted diseases are especially prone to take this form. Nocturnal fever is not especially fatal but it is long drawn out. Diurnal fever is longer still and sometimes leads to consumption. The seven-day fever is long-lasting but not fatal. The nine-day fever is still longer but not fatal. An exact tertian fever soon produces a crisis and is not fatal. The five-day fever is the worst of all, for when it comes on before consumption or when the patient be already consumptive, it is fatal.

25. Each of these fevers has its characteristics, both in the nature of the fever and the spacing of the paroxysms. For example, a continued fever in some cases rapidly attains its height and then the fever diminishes as the crisis is approached and is passed. In other cases it begins gently without producing obvious signs, increasing day by day paroxysmally until at the crisis it fairly shines out. In other fevers, the start is mild but the fever increases in paroxysms to its height and then persists until the crisis be reached and passed. These different signs may be displayed by any fever or sickness. Before deciding on treatment, you must also consider the patient's mode of life. There are also many other signs of importance to be considered in these conditions; some have already been described elsewhere, others await description. They must all be taken into account in deciding whether the patient will have a short or protracted illness, a fatal outcome or cure. Similarly these things will have to be considered in deciding what treatment to adopt and the nature, quantity and time of administration of medicaments.

26. Fevers attended by paroxysms at even numbers of days, reach their crisis also in an even number; if the paroxysms are on odd days, so is the crisis. The first period (of fever) in those maladies which reach the crisis in an even number of days is 4, 6, 8, 10, 14, 20, 24, 30, 40, 60, 80 or 120 days. If the crisis be reached in an odd number, then the first period lasts 3, 5, 7, 9, 11, 17, 21, 27 or 31 days. It must be noted that if a crisis occurs on any other day than those mentioned, there will be a relapse and also it may prove a fatal sign. One must pay attention to these days which have been specified in the course of a particular fever and realize that on them a crisis may take place leading to recovery or death, to improvement or to deterioration. In irregular fevers, quartans, five-, seven- and nine-day fevers, one must also take note of the periodicity with which the crises occur.

FOURTEEN CASES

(i)

Philiscus lived near the city wall. He took to his bed on the first day of his illness with high fever and sweating and passed an uneasy night.

On the second day all the symptoms became more pronounced, and later in the day his bowels were well opened following the administration of an enema. He spent a quiet night.

Third day: in the early morning and until midday he appeared afebrile: towards evening, a high fever with sweating, thirst, a parched tongue and he passed dark urine. Spent a restless night without sleeping and was quite out of his mind.

Fourth day: symptoms more pronounced; urine dark. An easier night; urine a better colour.

Fifth day: about midday a slight epistaxis of pure blood; urine not homogeneous but containing globular particles suspended in it, like semen, which did not settle. Following the giving of a suppository, passed small stools with flatulence. Night uneasy, short snatches of sleep, delirium, extremities all cold and could not be warmed, passed dark urine, slept a little towards daybreak, lost his voice, cold sweating, extremities livid.

About midday on the sixth day he died.

Throughout he took deep infrequent breaths, as if consciously controlling his breathing. The spleen was enlarged and presented as a round lump; cold sweats all through the illness. The paroxysms were on even days.

(ii)

Silenus lived on the flat ground near Evalcidas' place. He took a fever as the result of fatigue, drink and untimely exercise. He started with a pain in the loins, heaviness of the head and retraction of the neck.

On the first day, stools copious, bilious and not homogeneous; frothy and dark-coloured. Urine dark with a dark sediment; thirst, tongue dry; did not sleep that night.

Second day: high fever, stools more copious, thinner and frothy; urine dark. Passed a restless night, slight delirium.

Third day: all symptoms more pronounced; contraction of the hypochondrium on both sides extending as far as the navel, somewhat flabby underneath the contraction. Stools thin and somewhat dark in colour; urine cloudy and rather dark. No sleep that night, much talking, laughter, singing, could not be restrained.

Fourth day: condition unchanged.

Fifth day: stools unmixed, bilious, smooth and fatty; urine thin and clear; showed slight signs of understanding.

Sixth day: slight sweating about the head, extremities cold and livid, much tossing about, complicated with constipation and anuria, high fever.

Seventh day: lost his voice, extremities could no longer be warmed, anuria and retention of stools continued.

Eighth day: cold sweating all over, accompanied by spots. These were red, round and small like those of acne which did not go down. A thin copious stool, as if undigested, was passed with difficulty following a small enema. The urine was passed with pain and was pungent; extremities became slightly warm, periods of light sleep, signs of coma, loss of voice, urine thin and clear.

Ninth day: condition unchanged.

Tenth day: would not take drink, comatose, periods of light sleep; stools the same, passed a large quantity of rather thick urine which formed a white sediment like barley-meal on standing. Extremities again cold.

Eleventh day: he died.

From the beginning and throughout the illness he took deep infrequent breaths. Continuous pulsation of the hypochondrium. Age about twenty.

(iii)

Herophon suffered from a high fever. Stools small with tenesmus at first; afterwards he passed thin bilious matter rather frequently. He could not sleep, urine dark and thin.

Early on the fifth day, became deaf, all the symptoms were

more pronounced, the spleen became enlarged, the hypochondrium contracted; he passed a small quantity of dark matter from his bowels. He was delirious.

Sixth day: babbling at random, at night sweating, became cold, remained delirious.

Seventh day: became cold, thirsty, out of his mind. Regained control of his mind during the night and slept.

Eighth day: fever; the spleen was reduced in size and he was, wholly lucid. He felt a pain at first in the groin on the same side as the spleen, later on pains in the calves of both legs. Passed a comfortable night. Urine of better colour with a slight sediment.

Ninth day: sweating, the crisis was reached and the fever left him.

On the fifth day after this a relapse occurred. The spleen immediately enlarged; high fever, deafness again. On the third day of the relapse the spleen became reduced, the deafness less; pain in the legs; sweating during the night. A crisis was reached about the seventeenth day. There was no delirium during the relapse.

(iv)

In Thasos, the wife of Philinus, having given birth to a daughter fourteen days previously, the lochia being normal and the patient doing well, was taken ill with a fever accompanied by rigors. At first she felt a pain in the heart and in the right hypochondrium; pains in the genitalia; the lochia ceased. When a pessary was applied the pain in the perineum was eased, but the pains in the head, neck and loins remained. No sleep, extremities cold, thirst, belly dried up, passed small stools, urine thin and of bad colour at first.

On the sixth night, a long attack of delirium followed by lucidity.

Seventh day: thirst, small bilious dark-coloured stools.

Eighth day: further rigors, high fever, a large number of painful convulsions, much talking at random. An enema produced copious bilious stools. Sleep not possible.

Ninth day: convulsions.

Tenth day: slight recovery of senses.

Eleventh day: slept, remembered everything, but very soon became delirious again. Passed much urine spontaneously accompanied by frequent convulsions; the urine was thick and white, looking like urine with a sediment which has been stirred up, but when it was left standing a long time it did not in fact produce a sediment and resembled in colour and thickness the urine of cattle. I myself examined the urine.

About the fourteenth day, a throbbing throughout the body, a lot of talking, slight lucidity rapidly followed by renewed delirium.

About the seventeenth day she became speechless and died on the twentieth day.

(v)

The wife of Epicrates, who lived near the statue of the founder, was said to have had a violent shivering fit about the time of child-birth, and could not get warm. The severe symptoms continued on the next day.

On the third day she gave birth to a daughter and parturition was normal.

On the second day of the puerperium she had a high fever with pains in the heart and in the genitals which were eased by the application of a pessary. But she continued to suffer from pains in the head, neck and loins. Sleep was impossible. Her stools were small, thin, bilious and not homogeneous; urine thin and rather dark.

On the night of the sixth day of the fever she became delirious.

The symptoms became more pronounced on the seventh day; insomnia, delirium, thirst, dark-coloured bilious stools.

Eighth day: rigors occurred, she slept rather more.

Ninth day: no change.

Tenth day: painful aching in the legs, pain recurred in the heart, headache, no delirium, slept more, bowels constipated.

Eleventh day: passed a lot of urine of good colour which produced a sediment. Was rather better.

Fourteenth day: rigors, high fever.

Fifteenth day: vomited yellow bilious matter rather frequently, sweated and became feverish; at night high fever again, urine thick with a white sediment.

Sixteenth day: a paroxysm, restless night, no sleep, delirium.

Eighteenth day: thirst, tongue parched, no sleep, a lot of delirium, pains in the legs.

About the twentieth day, slight rigors early in the morning, coma, slept restfully, vomited a small quantity of bilious dark matter, deafness at night.

About the twenty-first day, a painful heaviness all down the left side; coughed up a small amount. Urine thick, cloudy and reddish; did not form a sediment when left standing. An improvement in other respects but she remained febrile. From the beginning of the illness the throat was painful and inflamed with the uvula retracted, and there was a pungent acrid salty discharge.

About the twenty-seventh day, no fever, a sediment in the urine, slight ache in the side.

About the thirty-first day the fever returned and the bowels were disordered, the stools bilious.

On the fortieth day she vomited a small quantity of bilious matter.

The final crisis and the end of the fever was reached on the eightieth day.

(vi)

Cleanactides, who lived on the hill above the temple of Heracles, was taken ill with an irregular fever. From the beginning he suffered from headache and pain in the left side; the rest of the body ached as it might from fatigue. The paroxysms of fever occurred in no regular sequence, but sometimes in one fashion, sometimes another. Sometimes there was sweating; sometimes not. Generally paroxysms were specially in evidence on the critical days.

About the twenty-fourth day he suffered from pain in the finger-tips and vomited, at first yellow bilious material, later rust-coloured matter. He vomited up everything.

About the thirtieth day he began to bleed from both nostrils and slight epistaxis continued until the crisis. He did not suffer at all from anorexia, thirst or insomnia. Urine was thin, but not of a bad colour.

About the fortieth day he passed reddish urine with a large amount of red sediment. His condition improved. Subsequently the nature of the urine was varied; sometimes it had a sediment, sometimes none.

On the sixtieth day the urine contained a lot of white smooth sediment. All the symptoms decreased and the fever left him; the urine again became thin but of a good colour.

On the seventieth day, fever followed by ten days' remission.

On the eightieth day, rigors and high fever; he sweated a lot, and the urine contained a red smooth sediment. Eventually the final crisis was reached.

(vii)

Meton suffered from a fever with a painful heaviness in the loins.

Second day: he took frequent drinks of water and his bowels were well opened.

Third day: heaviness in the head; the stools thin, bilious and reddish.

Fourth day: symptoms more pronounced; on two occasions he had an epistaxis from the right nostril. Passed a restless night; stools as on the third day; urine rather dark in colour and containing suspended particles which did not settle on standing.

Fifth day: a copious epistaxis from the left nostril of pure blood, sweating; the crisis was reached.

After the crisis, he had insomnia and delirium while his urine was thin and rather dark. He had his head bathed, slept and regained his wits. He did not relapse but he had many attacks of epistaxis following the crisis.

(viii)

Erasinus lived near the gully of Boötes. He was taken ill with fever after dinner and passed a disturbed night.

E

The first day was restful; was distressed during the night.

Second day: all symptoms more pronounced, delirium at night.

Third day: painful, much delirium.

Fourth day: worst of all so far; did not sleep at all at night. Visual hallucinations, delirium. These were followed by even more marked disturbances, feelings of fear and his illness was very severe.

Fifth day: in the early morning he became lucid and quite regained possession of his wits. But some time before noon he became mad and could not be restrained; extremities cold and somewhat livid. Suppression of urine. He died about sunset.

He had fever throughout the illness accompanied by sweating. The hypochondrium was distended and contracted only with pain. The urine was dark containing suspended globular particles which did not form a sediment on standing. His bowels remained open and he passed solid stools. Thirst throughout was not excessive. He had many convulsions accompanied by sweating about the time of death.

(ix)

Crito in Thasos had a violent pain in the foot which came on while walking; it started from the big toe. The same day he took to his bed with shivering, nausea and slight fever; at night he became delirious.

Second day: the whole foot became swollen; it was reddish about the ankle where there was some contraction and small black blisters appeared. He developed high fever and madness. He passed rather frequent unmixed bilious stools.

He died on the second day from the beginning of his illness.

(x)

The man from Clazomenae, who was dwelling near the well of Phrynichides, took a fever. From the beginning he had headache and aching pains in his neck and loins. Deafness was present from the start; sleep was impossible. High fever developed, the hypochondrium was distended but not excessively so, distension, tongue dry.

On the night of the fourth day he became delirious.

Fifth day: bad.

Sixth day: all symptoms more pronounced.

About the eleventh day a slight relief.

From the beginning of the illness until the fourteenth day the stools were thin, bile-stained and copious. Then the bowels became constipated. The urine throughout, although thin, was copious and of a good colour and contained scattered particles which did not settle.

About the sixteenth day he passed slightly thicker urine which formed a small amount of sediment. He became a little better and more lucid.

On the seventeenth day the urine became thin again and painful parotid swellings appeared. Sleep was impossible; he was delirious and suffered from pain in the legs.

On the twentieth day he attained the crisis and became afebrile; he did not sweat, became completely lucid.

About the twenty-seventh day he had a violent pain in the right hip which quickly ceased. The swellings near the ears neither suppurated nor resolved, but remained painful.

About the thirty-first day, diarrhoea started; the stools were very watery with some evidence of dysentery. He passed thick urine. The swellings by the ears went down.

On the fortieth day his right eye ached and his sight became impaired; this trouble passed off.

(xi)

The wife of Dromeades, having given birth to a daughter and progressing in all other respects normally, was seized by rigors on the second day, accompanied with high fever.

A pain started on the subsequent day in the hypochondrium; nausea and shivering supervened. She did not sleep on succeeding days and was distraught. Breathing deep and slow, each breath immediately drawn back again.

On the second day after the rigors, her stools were normal; the urine thick, white and cloudy, of the appearance of urine

with sediment which has been stirred up after standing a long
while. But in her case no sediment was formed. She did not
sleep at night.

Third day: about noon rigors, a high fever, urine as before,
pain in the hypochondrium, nausea. A restless night with
insomnia. Generalized cold sweats, but soon followed by
warmth again.

Fourth day: slight relief of the pain in the hypochondrium,
a heavy headache. Fell into a stupor; a slight epistaxis
occurred. Tongue dry, thirst. Urine little, thin and oily.
Slept a little.

Fifth day: thirst, nausea; character of urine unchanged,
constipated. About noon much delirium followed quickly by
a lucid phase. On going to stool she became comatose and
chilled, slept during the night but was delirious.

Early on the sixth day she suffered from rigors followed
quickly by fever and generalized sweating; the extremities
were cold and she was delirious with a slow rate of breathing.
After a little while convulsions supervened starting in the
head and death soon followed.

(xii)

A man dined when heated and drank too much. During
the night he vomited everything up; high fever, pain in the
right hypochondrium with a soft inflammation therein; a restless night. Urine at first was thick and red and did not sediment
when left to stand. Tongue dry but no excessive thirst.

Fourth day: high fever; generalized pain.

Fifth day: passed a large amount of smooth oily urine. High
fever.

Sixth day: towards evening, much delirium. Insomnia.

Seventh day: all symptoms more pronounced. Urine as
before; very talkative and could not be restrained. Following
an enema he passed a liquid disturbed stool containing worms.
A bad night; rigors in the early morning. High fever with
warm sweating, then appeared to lose the fever. He did not
sleep much and was chilled after sleeping. Expectoration. In

the evening much delirium and after a short while vomited a small amount of black bilious matter.

Ninth day: chilled, much delirious babbling, insomnia.

Tenth day: pains in the legs, all symptoms more pronounced, delirium.

Eleventh day: death.

(xiii)

A woman who lived on the sea-front was seized with a fever while in the third month of pregnancy. She was immediately seized with pains in the loins.

On the third day, pain in the head, neck and round about the right clavicle. Very shortly the tongue became unable to articulate and the right arm was paralysed following a convulsion as happens in hemiplegia. Her speech was delirious. A restless night with insomnia; the bowels were disordered and the stools were small, bilious and unmixed.

Fourth day: speech was indistinct but she was no longer paralysed, convulsions. Pains continued as before and there was a painful swelling near the hypochondrium. She did not sleep and was completely delirious. Bowels disordered; urine thin and not of a good colour.

Fifth day: high fever; pain in the hypochondrium, completely delirious. Stools bilious. At night she sweated and the fever left her.

Sixth day: lucid; a general improvement; pain persisted in the region of the left clavicle. Thirst, thin urine, insomnia.

Seventh day: trembling, fell into a stupor with slight delirium. Aching persisted about the clavicle and in the left upper arm, but in other respects her condition improved and she was fully lucid. The fever intermitted for three days.

On the eleventh day a relapse occurred with rigors and fever.

About the fourteenth day she vomited yellow bilious material rather frequently; sweating. Reached a crisis and the fever left her.

(xiv)

Melidia, who lay near the temple of Hera, began to suffer from violent headache and pain in the neck and chest. She was at once seized with a fever. There was some vaginal discharge. The pain from which she suffered was continuous.

Sixth day: fell into a coma, nausea, shivering, a rash appeared on the face, slightly delirious.

Seventh day: sweating. The fever declined but the pain remained. The fever returned; short snatches of sleep.

Urine was of good colour throughout but thin. The stools were thin, bilious and pungent, small in quantity, dark and offensive. The urine contained a white smooth sediment. Sweating took place. The final crisis was reached on the eleventh day.

EPIDEMICS, BOOK III

1. (i)

Pythion who lived near the temple of Earth suffered from twitching which began in the hands.

First day: high fever, delirium.

Second day: all symptoms more pronounced.

Third day: condition unchanged.

Fourth day: passed small, undigested, bilious stools.

Fifth day: all symptoms more pronounced, periods of light sleep, bowels constipated.

Sixth day: sputum not homogeneous and tinged red.

Seventh day: mouth distorted.

Eighth day: all symptoms more pronounced, fits of twitching continued. From the beginning of the illness until the eighth day, the urine was thin and pale, with cloudy matter in it.

Tenth day: sweated, sputum rather ripe, the crisis reached; urine rather thin about the time of the crisis. After the crisis, in fact forty days later, a peri-anal abscess formed which produced the symptom of strangury.

(ii)

Hermocrates, who lay near the new wall, took a fever. It started with a headache and pain in the loins. The hypochondrium was flabby and distended and the tongue was parched. He immediately became deaf, was unable to sleep, was thirsty but not excessively so, while the urine was thick and red and formed no sediment. There was some inflammatory matter in the stools.

Fifth day: passed thin urine which had particles suspended in it but which did not form a sediment; became delirious towards nightfall.

Sixth day: signs of jaundice; all symptoms more pronounced, not mentally lucid.

Seventh day: condition uneasy, urine thin as before. Condition remained more or less unchanged on the following days. About the eleventh day there was the appearance of general improvement but then coma supervened; he passed thicker reddish urine which was clear below. Slowly became lucid.

Fourteenth day: afebrile, no sweating, slept, fully lucid. Urine much as before. A relapse with fever around about the seventeenth day. This was followed by high fever on succeeding days; delirium, thin urine. A second crisis occurred on the twentieth day; became afebrile, no sweating. The whole time he suffered from loss of appetite. He was fully lucid, but was unable to converse. Tongue dry but no thirst. Slept a little, then comatose. About the twenty-fourth day there was a further rise of temperature with diarrhoea. On the following days high fever continued and his tongue was parched.

Twenty-seventh day: died.

The patient's deafness lasted throughout his illness; the urine was thick and red forming no sediment, or else thin and colourless with suspended particles in it. The patient also lost his sense of taste.

(iii)

A man who dwelt in the park of Delearces suffered for a long time from heaviness of the head and right temporal pain. For some reason he took a fever and went to bed.

Second day: a small flow of pure blood from the left nostril. Bowels well opened; urine thin and not homogeneous, containing small suspended particles like barley-meal or semen.

Third day: a high fever; stools dark, thin and frothy with a livid sediment. Patient became stuporous; going to stool caused discomfort. Urine had a livid somewhat sticky sediment.

Fourth day: vomited small quantities of yellow bilious matter and, after a while, a small quantity of rust-coloured material. There was a small haemorrhage of pure blood from the left side of the nose, stools and urine as before; sweating about the head and shoulders; spleen enlarged; pain in the region of the thigh; a rather flabby distension of the right hypochondrium; did not sleep at night; slight delirium.

Fifth day: stools larger, dark and frothy with a dark sediment; no sleep that night, delirium.

Sixth day: stools dark, oily, sticky and foul-smelling. Slept and was rather more lucid.

Seventh day: tongue dry, thirsty, did not sleep, delirious; urine thin, but not of a good colour.

Eighth day: stools small and dark, formed; slept and became lucid; thirsty, but not excessively so.

Ninth day: rigors supervened, a high fever, sweating, chilling, delirium, squint in the right eye; tongue dry, thirst, insomnia.

Tenth day: condition unchanged.

Eleventh day: became fully lucid, afebrile, slept; urine was thin about the time of the crisis. He remained afebrile for a period of two days but a relapse occurred on the fourteenth day, when he immediately became completely delirious and was sleepless all night.

Fifteenth day: urine muddy, resembling the appearance of urine which contains sediment after it is stirred up; a high fever, completely delirious, pain in the knees and calves. Passed dark stools after the application of a suppository.

Sixteenth day: urine thin with cloudy matter suspended in it; delirium.

Seventeenth day: in the morning the extremities were cold; he was wrapped up, had high fever, sweating all over; condition improved, became more lucid but not afebrile; thirsty, vomited small quantities of yellow bilious matter; passed stools which after a little became dark, small in quantity and thin. Urine was thin but not of good colour.

Eighteenth day: was not lucid; comatose.

Nineteenth day: condition unchanged.

Twentieth day: slept, was fully lucid, sweating, afebrile; not thirsty, urine thin.

Twenty-first day: slight delirium, somewhat thirsty, pain in the hypochondrium associated with palpitation in the umbilical region.

Twenty-fourth day: sediment in the urine; was fully lucid.

Twenty-seventh day: pain in the right hip, but in other

respects doing very well; sediment in the urine. About the
twenty-ninth day, pain in the right eye; urine thin. On the
fortieth day, passed frequent white stools containing mucus;
sweated much all over and reached the final crisis.

(iv)

At Thasos, Philistes had a headache for a long time and,
on falling into a state of stupor one day, took to his bed. As a
result of drinking, continuous fever occurred and the pain
became worse. It was at night that he first became hot.

First day: vomited small quantities of yellow bilious matter
at first, afterwards more which was rust-coloured. Bowels
were opened. An uneasy night.

Second day: deafness, high fever; the right hypochondrium
was contracted and scaphoid; urine thin, transparent and
having a small amount of suspended particles in it resembling
semen. He became mad about midday.

Third day: uneasy.

Fourth day: convulsions, a fit.

Fifth day: died in the morning.

(v)

Chaerion who lay at the house of Delias took a fever as
the result of drinking. At once his head began to feel heavy
and to ache; he had no sleep, bowels disordered with thin,
rather bilious stools.

Third day: high fever, twitching of the head, particularly of
the lower lip. After a while, rigor, convulsions, complete
delirium; passed an uneasy night.

Fourth day: quiet, slept a little, delirious.

Fifth day: condition bad, all symptoms more pronounced,
random babbling, an uneasy sleepless night.

Sixth day: condition unchanged.

Seventh day: rigors, high fever, sweating all over; the crisis
reached. Throughout his stools were bilious, small in quantity
and undigested. Urine thin, of poor colour and with a cloudy
substance suspended in it. About the eighth day he passed

urine of a better colour which had a small amount of white sediment; he became lucid and afebrile and there was an intermission. On the ninth day a relapse occurred.

Fourteenth day: high fever.

Sixteenth day: vomited bilious yellow matter rather frequently.

Seventeenth day: rigors, high fever, sweating; reached a crisis and the fever left him. After the relapse and then the crisis, the urine was of good colour with a sediment. Delirium was absent during the relapse.

Eighteenth day: slight rise in temperature, slight thirst, urine thin with a cloudy substance suspended in it; slight delirium.

Nineteenth day: afebrile, pain in the neck, sediment in the urine. The final crisis was reached on the twentieth day.

(vi)

The unmarried daughter of Euryanax took a fever. She suffered from no thirst throughout and did not take her food. Passed small stools; the urine thin, of small quantity and not of good colour. At the beginning of the fever she had pain around the anus. On the sixth day she became afebrile, did not sweat and reached a crisis. However, there was some slight suppuration about the anus, the abscess bursting about the time of the crisis. On the seventh day after the crisis, rigors occurred and there was slight fever with sweating. Subsequently she was always cold about the extremities. About the tenth day after the sweating occurred, she became delirious, but quickly recovered her lucidity again. They said it was through eating grapes. After an intermission of twelve days, she again became quite delirious, the bowels were disordered, the stools being bilious, unmixed, small in quantity, thin and pungent. The stools were passed frequently. She died on the seventh day following the last attack of her illness and a rash was present throughout, while the uvula was retracted. Fluxes were present, small and acrid. Although she had a cough it was unproductive. She had no appetite the whole time, nor did she wish for anything. She had no thirst and drank nothing worth mentioning. She was silent and would not talk. She was depressed and despaired of herself. There was also some sign of an inherited tendency to consumption.

(vii)

The woman who suffered from sore throat, who lived near Aristion's place, started first with her voice becoming indistinct. Her tongue was red and parched.

First day: shivering; became febrile.

Third day: rigor, high fever; a hard reddish swelling on either side of the neck down to the chest, extremities cold and livid, respiration superficial. What she drank was regurgitated through the nostrils and she was unable to swallow. Stools and urine suppressed.

Fourth day: all symptoms more pronounced.

Fifth day: died.

(viii)

The lad who lay by the Liars' Market took a fever as the result of exhaustion, having exerted himself by running more than he was accustomed.

First day: bowels disordered with copious thin bilious stools; urine thin, rather dark; insomnia, thirst.

Second day: all symptoms more pronounced; stools more copious and unhealthy. No sleep; his mind was disordered; slight sweating.

Third day: uneasy, thirst, nausea, much tossing about, distress, delirium, extremities cold and livid; a somewhat flabby bilateral distension of the hypochondrium.

Fourth day: no sleep; condition deteriorated.

Seventh day: died.

Age about twenty.

(ix)

The woman at the house of Tisamenus was taken to her bed feeling very ill with symptoms suggesting an attack of ileus. Much vomiting; she could keep neither food nor drink down. Pain in the hypochondrium; also pain lower down in the belly proper. Constant colic. No thirst. Became warm, but the extremities remained cold throughout; nausea; insomnia. Urine small in quantity and thin. Stools raw, thin and small. It was impossible to do anything to help her; she died.

(x)

A woman of the household of Pantimides took a fever the first day after a miscarriage. Tongue was parched; thirst, nausea and insomnia, bowels disordered, the stools being thin, copious and raw.

Second day: rigors, high fever, much purgation; did not sleep.

Third day: pains more intense.

Fourth day: became delirious.

Seventh day: died.

The bowels were relaxed throughout, the stools being watery, thin, raw and voluminous; urine little and thin.

(xi)

Another case of miscarriage about the fifth month resulted in Hicetas' wife taking a fever. To begin with she was comatose but later became wakeful and suffered from pain in the loins and heaviness of the head.

Second day: bowels disordered with small, thin stools, at first unmixed.

Third day: worse; did not sleep at night.

Fourth day: became delirious and suffered from fears and from depression. Squint in the right eye; a small amount of cold sweating about the head. Extremities cold.

Fifth day: all symptoms more pronounced; much delirious talking, but she soon became lucid again. No thirst, insomnia; the stools were large in quantity, and unfavourable throughout; urine little in quantity, thin and rather dark. Extremities cold and somewhat livid.

Sixth day: no change.

Seventh day: death.

(xii)

A woman who lay near the Liars' Market, having given birth to a first-born male child after a difficult labour, took a fever. To start with she suffered from thirst, nausea and a slight ache in the heart; her tongue was parched and the bowels were disordered, her stools being thin and small. She did not sleep.

Second day: slight rigors, a high fever, a small amount of cold sweating about the head.

Third day: distressed; passed a large quantity of raw thin stools.

Fourth day: rigors, all symptoms more pronounced. Insomnia.

Fifth day: distressed.

Sixth day: no change; passed a large quantity of liquid stools.

Seventh day: rigors, high fever, thirst, much tossing about. Towards evening, cold sweating all over and became chilled; the extremities were cold and did not get warm again. Further rigors during the night; extremities still would not get warm; no sleep and some delirium which quickly passed off.

Eighth day: about noon, she became warm, thirsty and comatose; nausea, vomited a small quantity of yellowish bile-stained material. An uneasy night without sleep. Frequently unconsciously incontinent of large quantities of urine.

Ninth day: all symptoms abated; comatose. In the afternoon had rigors, vomited a small amount of bilious material.

Tenth day: rigor, fever increased in a paroxysm; had no sleep at all. Early in the morning she passed a large quantity of urine which did not show a sediment. Extremities became warm.

Eleventh day: vomited bilious rust-coloured material. Shortly afterwards, she had rigors and the extremities became cold again. Towards evening, sweating, rigors and much vomiting; a distressed night.

Twelfth day: vomited much dark, foul-smelling matter; much sobbing, a distressing thirst.

Thirteenth day: vomited much dark foul-smelling matter; rigor. About midday she lost her voice.

Fourteenth day: epistaxis. Death.

This patient throughout had relaxed bowels and shivery attacks; age about seventeen.

2. The year was rainy and southerly; throughout there was no wind. Droughts having occurred immediately before, about the rising of Arcturus, there was much rain accompanied by southerly winds. The autumn was overcast and cloudy with a very heavy rainfall. The winter was southerly and wet; mild after the solstice. Much later, near the equinox, belated storms occurred and, right at the equinox, a spell of northerly winds bringing snow but this did not last long. The spring again was southerly and calm; rainfall continued to be heavy until the rising of the Dog Star. The summer was fine and warm, and there were periods of stifling heat. The etesian winds blew feebly and at scattered intervals. Again about the rising of Arcturus, northerly winds brought much rain.

The whole year then being southerly, wet and mild, health was good during the winter, except in the case of the consumptive, about whom I shall write.

3. Early in the spring, just at the time the cold snaps occurred, there was a lot of severe erysipelas; in some cases from some obvious cause, but in others from none. Many cases proved fatal and many had a painful throat. The symptoms were a weakened voice, *causus* accompanied by brain fever, aphthae in the mouth, tumours in the pudendal region, ophthalmia, carbuncles, disorders of the bowels, anorexia, sometimes thirst, abnormalities of the urine which was abundant and bad. The patients were mainly comatose, but again there were periods of wakefulness. Very often there was no crisis or it was attained with difficulty. There was also dropsy and much consumption. Such were the epidemic diseases; the sick fell into the classes given above, and many of them died. The course of the various diseases was as follows.

4. In many cases erysipelas occurred which spread all over the body on any chance happening and especially following a

slight wound; those about sixty years of age were particularly liable to it in the head if any wound there were slightly neglected. Many cases, too, under treatment suffered from extensive inflammation, the erysipelas spreading rapidly in all directions. In the majority of cases abscessions turned to collections of pus. There was much destruction of flesh, sinews and bones. The fluid which formed in the abscess was not like (ordinary) pus, but a different sort of morbid fluid, being both copious and varied. In those cases where something of this sort affected the head, the whole head would become bald including the beard; the bones became thin and formed sequestra, while there was a discharge at many points.

These symptoms occurred both with and without fever. They were more frightening than serious, for when the disease resulted in the formation of a localized collection of pus, or some similar ripe condition, the majority recovered. On the other hand, when the inflammation and the erysipelas departed without causing such abscess formation, many sufferers died. Much the same happened if it wandered off to any other part of the body, for many had the whole arm or forearm waste away. Those whose sides were attacked, suffered harm in some part either in front or at the back of the body. In some cases, the whole thigh or the calf became thin and the whole foot too. The worst of all was if the disease attacked the pubes and private parts.

All these things happened as the result of a wound or of some obvious cause. But in many other cases it accompanied, preceded or followed fevers. In these cases, whenever localization took place with the formation of a collection of pus, or an opportune disturbance of the bowels, or favourable urine was passed, this resolved the disease. But when none of these symptoms occurred and the disease departed without giving a sign, it was fatal. By far the largest number of cases of erysipelas occurred in the spring; but it continued throughout the summer and on into the autumn.

5. Some people were very ill with pharyngeal swellings, inflammation of the tongue and abscesses in connection with the teeth.

A common sign at the onset, not only of consumption, but also in cases of *causus* and brain-fever, was a weakening and choking of the voice.

6. Cases of *causus* and brain-fever began early in the spring after the cold spells had passed, and many people were taken ill at that time. In these cases, the disease was acute and liable to prove fatal. The symptoms found in *causus* were as follows. To start with, the patients were comatose and nauseated, shivering and with high fever, but they were neither excessively thirsty nor delirious. Slight epistaxis occurred. In the majority of cases, the paroxysms took place on even days, and about the time of these paroxysms, there was loss of memory, exhaustion and loss of voice. The feet and hands were rather cold all the time but especially so at the paroxysms. Subsequently, the patients would get warm again slowly, but not thoroughly; they also became lucid and talked. They were also afflicted with a continuous coma but something that differed from sleep, or with a painful insomnia.

In most of these cases, the bowels were disordered, the stools being thin, raw and copious. The urine was copious too and thin, but giving none of the signs of crisis, nor any other helpful sign. In fact, those who were then attacked showed no crisis at all; there was no beneficient haemorrhage nor did critical abscess-formation of the usual sort occur. Many died after no fixed interval, but just as matters chanced; some at the crisis, some after a long period of aphonia, some in bouts of sweating. These were the symptoms in the fatal cases, but they were much the same in brain-fever. All these cases showed a complete absence of the symptoms of thirst; nor did any of those with brain-fever go mad as in other cases, but they perished with their heads weighed down by a growing stupor.

7. There were also other fevers which I shall describe. Many had aphthae and ulcers in the mouth; many had discharges around the pudendal area; while sores and tumours both external and internal occurred, some about the groin. Moist ophthalmia occurred which was both chronic and painful. Excrescence on the eyelids, both internal and external,

F

occurred and, in many cases, impaired the vision: the name 'figs' is given to these. There were many cases of growth on other ulcers and on the pudenda. Carbuncles were common during the summer and other septic lesions and large pustules. Many suffered from extensive herpetic lesions.

8. Frequent and dangerous disorders affecting the belly were common. First, many had distressing tenesmus; most of these were children, including all below the age of puberty, and most of these died. Many had enteritis or dysentery, but in these cases without overmuch distress. In some cases the stools were bilious, fatty, thin and watery. In many cases this was so at the inception of the disease, both with and without fever. Painful colic and malignant flatulent colic also occurred; in these going to stool did not relieve the pains, the stools being such that much remained within the bowel after attempted evacuation. This condition responded only with difficulty to medicines, and in most cases purgatives did additional harm. Many of those with this complaint perished soon; others lasted rather longer.

To sum up, whether their illnesses were long or short, all who suffered from disease of the belly were specially likely to die, for disease of the belly was a contributory factor in all the fatal cases.

9. In addition to all the previously mentioned symptoms, all suffered from anorexia, and that to an extent which I have never previously encountered. Those just described were especially affected, and particularly the hopeless cases both in this group and in the others mentioned. Some had a thirst, but not all. Those who had fevers or one of the other diseases had an intemperate thirst in no case, but they would take as much or as little to drink as you wished.

10. The amount of urine passed was great; it was not proportional to the amount drunk but considerably in excess. The urine which was passed was also markedly bad, for it possessed neither thickness nor ripeness. In most cases these signs signified some wasting and disorder of the bowels with pain and no crisis.

11. Those who suffered from brain-fever and *causus* were

particularly liable to become comatose, but this also occurred as an additional symptom in the other diseases in all the most serious cases, provided they were accompanied by fever. Throughout, most patients suffered either from deep coma or had only short periods of light sleep.

12. Many other types of fever were epidemic: tertians, quartans, nocturnal fevers, continued fevers, long fevers, irregular fevers, fever accompanied by nausea, and unstable fevers. All these were accompanied by much disturbance; the bowels were disordered and the patients were liable to shivering attacks. Sweating took place but did not mark the crisis; the condition of the urine has been described. In most of these cases, the illness was prolonged, for even when abscess formation did occur, it did not bring about a crisis in the way usual with other cases. In general, the diseases reached a crisis with difficulty, or there was no crisis and the illness remained chronic; this was specially the case with these people. A few of them had a crisis about the eightieth day, but in most the disease departed at no fixed time. A few died of dropsy without having been confined to their beds. Many were troubled with swellings in addition to their other diseases; especially the consumptive.

13. But it was consumption which proved the most widespread and the most serious complaint and this was responsible for most of the deaths. In many cases it began during the winter and, though many took to their beds, some of those who were ill did not do so. By early spring, most of those who had taken to their beds had died. In other cases, the cough, although it did not go away altogether, was less troublesome during the summer. Towards autumn, all took to their beds and many died. Of these, the majority had had a long illness.

In most cases, the illness started with sudden deterioration. The symptoms were: frequent shivering attacks, often high continued fever, much untimely sweating although the patients remained cold throughout, and much chilling so that it was difficult to get them warm again. Their bowels were inconstant, constipation rapidly giving way to diarrhoea, while near the end, diarrhoea was violent in all cases. The lungs were evacuated downwards; although the urine was large in quantity it was unfavourable. Wasting was pernicious. Coughing continued throughout the illness, and it was common for patients to bring up large amounts of ripe moist sputum, without excessive pain. But even in the cases where there was pain, the process of ridding the lungs from matter took place quite mildly. The pharynx was not painful, nor did salty humours cause any trouble. There were however copious discharges from the head of sticky, white, moist and frothy material. These patients, like those already described above, suffered by far the greatest harm from their loss of appetite. They would not even take fluid nourishment, but remained without thirst. As death approached, they showed heaviness of the body, coma, swelling becoming dropsical, shivering and delirium.

14. The appearance which characterizes consumptives is a smoothness of the skin, slight pallor, freckles, a slight flush, sparkling eyes, white sputum and winging of the shoulder-blades. The signs were the same in women too. They also show melancholy and suffused cheeks.

Causus, brain-fever and dysentery might follow upon these symptoms. The young, who were liable to phlegm, suffered from tenesmus. Those subject to bitter bile had long-lasting diarrhoea and acrid, greasy stools.

15. In all the cases so far described, the spring was the worst time and most of the deaths occurred then; the summer was the easiest time and few died then. Deaths occurred again during the autumn and under the Pleiads, in most cases on the fourth day. It seems to me that a normal summer is beneficial. For the coming of winter terminates summer diseases, and the coming of summer shifts winter diseases. All the same, considered by itself, the summer in question was not a settled one; for it suddenly turned hot, southerly and windless, but this was beneficial by being such a change from the previous weather.

SIXTEEN CASES

17.[1] (i)

At Thasos, the man from Paros who lay beyond the temple of Artemis took a high fever, at first of the continued type like that of *causus*, with thirst. At first he was comatose, then wakeful again; the bowels were disordered at first and the urine thin.

Sixth day: passed oily urine; delirious.

Seventh day: all symptoms more pronounced; did not sleep at all, urine unchanged, mind disordered. The stools were bilious and greasy.

Eighth day: slight epistaxis; vomited a small quantity of rust-coloured matter. Small amount of sleep.

Ninth day: no change.

Tenth day: all symptoms showed a decrease in severity.

Eleventh day: sweated all over and became chilled, but quickly got warm again.

Fourteenth day: high fever, stools bilious, thin and copious; urine contained suspended matter. Delirium.

Seventeenth day: distressed, for the patient was sleepless and the fever increased.

Twentieth day: sweating all over, afebrile, stools bilious, no appetite, comatose.

Twenty-fourth day: a relapse.

Thirty-fourth day: afebrile; bowels not constipated. Temperature rose again.

Fortieth day: afebrile, bowels constipated for a short while, no appetite, slight fever returned and was, throughout, irregular; at times he was afebrile, at others not. Any remission and improvement was followed quickly by a relapse. He took but little food and that poor stuff. He slept badly and showed delirium about the time of the relapses. At these times he passed thicker urine, but it was disturbed and bad. The bowels were sometimes constipated, sometimes relaxed. Slight fever continued throughout, and the stools were thin and copious.

[1] Section 16 appears to be an interpolation and is omitted.

Died in 120 days.

In this case, the bowels from the first day were either loose with copious bilious stools, or he passed frothy undigested constipated stools. The urine was bad throughout. He was comatose for the most part, but he could not sleep when in pain. At no time did he have any appetite.

(ii)

At Thasos, a woman who lay near the cold spring gave birth to a daughter. The lochia were withheld and on the third day she had a high fever with shivering. For a long while before delivery she had been febrile, had kept to her bed and suffered from anorexia. After the preliminary rigor, fever was high and continued and accompanied by shivering. On the eighth day and subsequent days there was much delirium, but she quickly became lucid again. The bowels were disordered and she passed thin copious stools like watery bile. No thirst.

Eleventh day: was both lucid and comatose. Passed much thin dark urine. Sleepless.

Twentieth day: slight chilling but quickly became warm again; slight delirious talking, insomnia. No change in the condition of the bowels; much watery urine.

Twenty-seventh day: afebrile, bowels constipated. Not long afterwards she had a violent pain in the right hip which lasted a long time. Fevers followed again; urine watery.

Fortieth day: pain in the hip lessened, but she had continued moist cough. Bowels constipated, no appetite, no change in the urine. The fever showed no remission generally, but exacerbation occurred in no regular pattern.

Sixtieth day: the cough ceased without any signs, for there was no ripening of the sputum nor any of the other signs of localization. The mandible was in spasm and protruded to the right and the patient comatose; then followed delirious talking quickly giving way to lucidity. She was obstinately averse to food. The jaw became normal again, but she continued to pass small quantities of bilious matter in the stools. The fever was higher and was accompanied by shivering. The voice was lost in subsequent days but was regained.

Died on the eighteenth day.

In this case the urine was dark, thin and watery throughout. Coma set in and there was loss of appetite, despondency, insomnia, fits of anger and agitation associated with a melancholy disposition.

(iii)

At Thasos, Pythion, who lay beyond the temple of Heracles, had a violent rigor and high fever as the result of strain, exhaustion and insufficient attention to his diet. Tongue parched, he was thirsty and bilious and did not sleep. Urine rather dark containing suspended matter which did not settle.

Second day: about midday, chilling of the extremities, particularly about the hands and head, showed both aphasia and aphonia, and he also was dyspnoeic for a long time. Then he became warm again and thirsty. A quiet night; slight sweating about the head.

Third day: quiet. Late in the day, about sunset, slight chilling, nausea, disturbed bowels followed by an uneasy sleepless night. Passed a small constipated stool.

Fourth day: morning quiet. About midday, all symptoms more pronounced; chilled, aphasia, aphonia became worse. After a while he became warm again and passed dark urine containing suspended matter. A quiet night; slept.

Fifth day: seemed to improve, but there was a painful heaviness in the belly. Thirsty. An uneasy night.

Sixth day: morning quiet. In the evening the pains were more severe and paroxysmal. The bowels were well opened late at night after an enema. Slept during the night.

Seventh day: nausea, somewhat distressed. Passed oily urine. Much disturbed during the night, random talking, no sleep.

Eighth day: slept a little in the morning, but soon became chilly with loss of voice. Respiration was superficial and shallow, late at night he became warm again, but delirious. A slight improvement took place towards daybreak. Stools unmixed, small and bilious.

Ninth day: comatose; nauseated whenever he woke. No

excessive thirst. About sunset he became distressed, talked at random and this was followed by a bad night.

Tenth day: in the morning, he lost his voice, became very chilled, had high fever with much sweating and died.

In this case the distress was marked on the even days.

(iv)

A patient with brain-fever took to his bed on the first day of the illness and vomited much rust-coloured thin matter. He had severe fever accompanied by shivering and continuous sweating of the whole body. There was a painful heaviness of the head and neck. The urine was thin and contained a small amount of scattered particles suspended in it, but did not sediment. He passed a large single stool, became delirious and did not sleep.

Second day: he was voiceless in the morning; fever high, sweating without remission. The whole body throbbed and convulsions occurred during the night.

Third day: all symptoms more pronounced.

Fourth day: died.

(v)

At Larisa, a bald man suddenly had a pain in the right thigh. No treatment which he received did him any good.

First day: high fever of *causus* type, did not tremble, but the pain continued.

Second day: pains in the thigh were relieved, but the fever increased. The patient became somewhat distressed and did not sleep; the extremities were cold. He passed a lot of urine but this was not of a favourable kind.

Third day: the pain in the thigh ceased. His mind became unhinged and there was much disturbance and tossing about.

Fourth day: died about noon.

(vi)

At Abdera, Pericles took a high fever of continued type, accompanied by distress. He had much thirst, was nauseated and could not keep liquids down. He had splenomegaly and headache.

First day: epistaxis from the left nostril; the fever however increased considerably. He passed much cloudy white urine which did not sediment on standing.

Second day: all symptoms more pronounced. The urine however was thick and settled more. The nausea was less severe and the patient slept.

Third day: the fever became less and he passed a large quantity of ripe urine with a lot of sediment. A quiet night.

Fourth day: about noon he had a warm sweat involving the whole body, the fever left him and he reached the crisis. There was no relapse.

(vii)

A girl who lay at a house on the Sacred Way at Abdera took a fever of the *causus* type. She complained of thirst and was wakeful. Menstruation took place for the first time.

Sixth day: much nausea, redness and shivering; she was distraught.

Seventh day: no change. The urine, though thin, was of good colour and there was no trouble with the bowels.

Eighth day: deafness supervened, with high fever, insomnia, nausea and shivering. She became lucid. Urine the same.

Ninth day: no change, nor on the following days. The deafness persisted.

Fourteenth day: mind disordered; the fever became less.

Seventeenth day: a large epistaxis; the deafness became slightly less. Nausea and deafness was present on the following days as well as some delirium.

Twentieth day: pain in the feet and deafness. The delirium ceased and there was a slight nose-bleed and sweating; afebrile.

Twenty-fourth day: the fever returned and she was deaf again. The pain in the feet continued and her mind was wandering.

Twenty-seventh day: severe sweating and became afebrile. The deafness cleared up and, although pain in the feet remained, in other respects the final crisis was reached.

(viii)

Anaxion, who lay near the Thracian Gates at Abdera, took a high fever. There was continuous aching in the right side and a dry cough, but no spitting in the first few days. He suffered from thirst and insomnia, but the urine was copious, thin and of good colour.

Sixth day: delirium. No improvement as the result of warm fomentations.

Seventh day: distressed as the fever increased. The pain did not decrease, cough was troublesome and breathing difficult.

Eighth day: I bled him at the elbow; there was a large flow of blood as there should be. The pain decreased but the dry cough continued.

Eleventh day: the fever decreased. There was slight sweating about the head while the cough and the sputum from the lungs were moister.

Seventeenth day: began to expectorate a small quantity of ripe sputum and his condition improved.

Twentieth day: sweated and became afebrile. After the crisis he was thirsty and the matter evacuated from the lungs was not good.

Twenty-seventh day: the fever returned and, with coughing, he brought up much ripe matter. A large white sediment in the urine. His thirst was lost and his respiration became normal.

Thirty-fourth day: sweated all over; became afebrile. A complete crisis.

(ix)

Heropythus at Abdera had a headache; he remained up for a while but eventually went to bed with it. He lived near the upper high-road. He showed a fever of the *causus* type. At first he vomited much bilious matter and suffered from thirst and much distress. His urine was thin and dark; sometimes, but not always, it contained suspended matter. An uneasy night. The fever showed paroxysms at varying intervals, for the most part quite irregular.

About the fourteenth day, he complained of deafness and the fever increased; the urine remained as before.

Twentieth and following days: much delirium.

Fortieth day: a large epistaxis and became more lucid. The deafness was still present but was less severe. The fever abated. Small epistaxes occurred frequently on the following days.

About the sixtieth day the haemorrhages stopped but there was a violent ache in the right hip and the fever increased again. A little later, there was pain involving all the lower part of the body. It so happened that either the temperature was up and the deafness worse, or these two symptoms abated while the pain in the lower part of the body and about the hips became worse.

From the eightieth day onwards all the symptoms decreased, although none entirely disappeared. He passed urine of good colour with more sediment.

About the hundredth day, there was disorder of the bowels with the passage of copious bilious stools. This went on to a considerable extent for not a little while. The signs of dysentery, accompanied by pain, were associated with an easing off of the other symptoms. Generally speaking, the fever departed and the deafness ceased.

A final crisis took place on the 120th day.

(x)

Nicodemus took a fever at Abdera as the result of sexual indulgence and drinking. To start with he suffered from nausea and cardalgia, thirst and a parched tongue. His urine was thin and dark.

Second day: paroxysms of fever, shivering, nausea; no sleep. Vomited yellow bilious matter. Urine as before. A quiet night and he slept.

Third day: a general remission and improvement. About sunset he became somewhat distressed again and passed an uneasy night.

Fourth day: a rigor, much fever and pains all over. Urine thin containing suspended matter. Night again quiet.

Fifth day: all symptoms continued but were less pronounced.

Sixth day: pain all over as before; the urine contained suspended matter. Delirium.

Seventh day: improved.

Eighth day: all other symptoms abated.

Tenth and following days: the pains continued but were all less acute. The paroxysms and pains in this case were throughout more pronounced on the even days of the illness.

Twentieth day: passed white urine which, although thick, did not form a sediment on standing. Much sweating; appeared to become afebrile but again became warm in the evening with pains as before, shivering, thirst and slight delirium.

Twenty-fourth day: passed much white urine which contained a large quantity of sediment. Sweated all over profusely, the sweat being warm. Became afebrile as the crisis was passed.

(xi)

A woman at Thasos became morose as the result of a justifiable grief, and although she did not take to her bed, she suffered from insomnia, anorexia, thirst and nausea. She lived on the level ground near Pylades' place.

Early on the night of the first day, she complained of fears and talked much; she showed despondency and a very slight fever. In the morning she had many convulsions; when the convulsions had for the most part ceased, she talked at random and used foul language. Many intense and continuous pains.

Second day: condition unchanged; no sleep and the fever higher.

Third day: the convulsions ceased but lethargy and coma supervened followed by a return to consciousness, when she leapt up and could not be restrained. There was much random talking and high fever. That night she sweated profusely all over with warm sweat. She became afebrile and slept becoming quite lucid and reaching the crisis.

About the third day, the urine was dark and thin, and contained suspended matter, for the most part round particles, which did not sediment. About the time of the crisis, a copious menstrual discharge took place.

(xii)

A girl at Larisa took a high fever of the *causus* type. She had insomnia and thirst while her tongue was dry and smoke-coloured. The urine was of good colour but thin.

Second day: distressed; did not sleep.

Third day: the stools were bulky, watery and greenish. On the following days stools of similar character were passed without distress.

Fourth day: passed a small quantity of thin urine which contained suspended matter which did not settle. Delirium during the night.

Sixth day: a violent and copious epistaxis. Shivering was followed by profuse hot sweating all over; she became afebrile and reached the crisis.

She menstruated for the first time during this illness, while the fever was still present, but after the crisis. She was only a girl. Throughout, she suffered from nausea, shivering, a flushed face, aching eyes and heaviness of the head. In this case there was no relapse but a single crisis. The distress was experienced on the even days.

(xiii)

Apollonius at Abdera suffered for a long time without taking to his bed. He had an enlarged abdomen and a pain in the region of the liver to which he had become accustomed, for he became jaundiced, flatulent and of pallid complexion.

As a result of eating beef and drinking cows' milk, he developed what was a slight fever at first and went to bed. He got much worse through taking a large amount of milk, both boiled and cold, both goats' and sheep's, and by taking a generally bad diet. For the fever increased and he passed nothing worth mentioning in the stools of the food he took. He passed little urine and that was thin. He was unable to sleep.

He then became badly distended, suffered from thirst and became comatose. There was swelling, accompanied by an aching pain in the right hypochondrium. All the extremities were somewhat cold. He began talking at random, showed loss of memory in anything he said, and became disorientated.

About the fourteenth day from the time he took to his bed he had rigors, his temperature rose and he went out of his mind; there was shouting, disturbance and much talking, then he settled down again and relapsed into coma. Subsequently his bowels were upset, the stools being copious, bilious, raw and unmixed. The urine was dark, small in quantity and thin. There was much distress. The excreta were not always the same; sometimes they were small in quantity and dark and rust-coloured, or they were greasy, raw and pungent. At times too he seemed to pass milky substances.

About the twenty-fourth day he was more comfortable; in other respects the symptoms were unchanged, but he became slightly lucid. He could remember nothing from the time he took to his bed. Shortly afterwards, his mind was again disordered and there was a general tendency to deteriorate.

About the thirtieth day he had high fever, copious thin stools and delirium. Extremities cold; aphonia.

Thirty-fourth day: died.

Throughout this case, from the time I knew of it, the bowels were disordered and the urine was thin and dark; the patient also suffered from coma, insomnia and cold extremities, and he was delirious throughout.

(xiv)

At Cyzicus, a woman gave birth to twin girls; the labour was difficult and the lochia abnormal.

On the first day, there was high fever with shivering, and heaviness and aching of the head and neck. She was sleepless from the start and she was silent, scowling and disobedient. Urine thin and of bad colour, thirst, nausea for the most part, diarrhoea and constipation succeeding each other at no fixed intervals.

Sixth day: much random talking during the night; no sleep.

About the eleventh day went mad and then became lucid again; urine dark, thin and then, after an interval, oily. The bowels were disturbed, the stools being large in quantity and thin in consistency.

Fourteenth day: many convulsions, extremities cold, still no trace of lucidity, suppression of urine.

Sixteenth day: aphonia.

Seventeenth day: died.

(xv)

At Thasos the wife of Delearces, who lay on the level ground, took a high fever with shivering as the result of grief. From the start she used to wrap herself up, always remaining silent while she groped about, scratching and plucking out hair, and alternately wept and laughed. She did not sleep. She remained constipated even when the bowels were stimulated. She drank a little when reminded to do so; the urine was thin and small in quantity. Fever was slight to the touch; the extremities were chilly.

Ninth day: much random talking, but subsequently she quietened down and fell silent.

Fourteenth day: respiration infrequent; deep for a while and then the breaths would be short.

Seventeenth day: the bowels were stimulated and disordered stools were passed giving way to the actual liquid drunk, nothing being retained. She was insensible to everything. Skin taut and dry.

Twentieth day: much talking and then quietened down again; aphonia, respiration in short breaths.

Twenty-first day: died.

Throughout this case respiration was intermittent, and deep. She was insensible to everything, always kept herself wrapped up and either talked at random or kept silence.

(xvi)

At Meliboea, a young man who had been running a temperature for a long time as the result of drinking and much sexual indulgence, took to his bed. His symptoms were shivering, nausea, insomnia and lack of thirst.

On the first day, his bowels passed a large quantity of solid faeces accompanied by much fluid. On the following days he passed a large quantity of watery, greenish stools. His urine was thin and small in quantity, and of bad colour. Respiration at long intervals and deep after a while. There was a somewhat flabby distension of the upper part of the abdomen extending laterally towards the flanks. Palpitation of the heart was continuous throughout. He passed oily urine.

Tenth day: was delirious without excitement, being well-behaved and silent. Skin dry and taut. Stools either copious and thin, or bilious and greasy.

Fourteenth day: all symptoms more pronounced. Delirium with much talking at random.

Twentieth day: went mad, much tossing about, passed no urine, kept down a small amount of fluid.

Twenty-fourth day: died.

THE SCIENCE OF MEDICINE

This spirited defence of Medicine is a remarkable document of an age when there were no precautions against unqualified practitioners, and all physicians were exposed to charges of charlatanry. The title is often rendered 'The Art', but this gives the wrong impression, for it is the writer's main contention that Medicine is an exact science, not an undefinable art.

1. There are men who have made a business of abusing the sciences and, although they would not confess it themselves, their aim nevertheless is simply to display their own knowledge. But it seems to me that it is the aim and function of an intelligent mind to make new discoveries in whatever field such investigations may be useful, and also to bring to completion tasks that are but half-finished. On the other hand, a desire to belittle by abuse the scientific discoveries of others and to slander the discoveries of the learned to the illiterate, rather than to offer constructive criticism, is not so much the aim and function of an intelligent mind, as a proof of warped character and want of skill. Those who have the ambition to be scientists but not the necessary ability are equipped for the malicious habit of slandering their neighbours' work if it be right, or of censuring it if it be wrong. In other sciences, let those who can stop their enemies, each in his own subject. This thesis aims at answering the opponents of the science of medicine with a boldness to condemn based upon a sound knowledge of the subject it defends and upon the strength of trained judgement.

2. It appears to me that there is no science which has no basis in fact. It would be absurd to suppose something that exists non-existent. For what property of a non-existent thing could anyone point to as a proof of its existence? If it were possible to see what has no substance, just as we see what does exist, then one could no longer call such a thing non-existent because it would then appear alike to the eye and the mind

existent. But may not the truth be something like this; what exists is always visible and recognizable, and what does not exist is neither visible nor recognizable? The activities of the sciences that are taught are things that can be seen and there is none that is not visible in one form or another. I at least am of the opinion that it is from the visible forms of things that they take their names. It is absurd to suppose that forms spring from names; that were impossible since names are adopted by convention, whereas forms are not invented but are characteristic of those things from which they spring.

3. If some of my readers have not sufficiently grasped the argument, it may be explained more clearly in other words. Let us consider the science of medicine, since that is my own subject, by way of illustration. First of all I would define medicine as the complete removal of the distress of the sick, the alleviation of the more violent diseases and the refusal to undertake to cure cases in which the disease has already won the mastery, knowing that everything is not possible to medicine. It is my intention to prove that medicine does accomplish these things and is ever capable of doing them. And as I describe the science I shall at the same time disprove the arguments of her traducers, whatever way each prides himself on his attack.

4. My first premise is one that everyone accepts; for it is admitted that some who have received medical attention have been restored to health. But the fact that everyone is not cured is reckoned an argument against the science, while those who recover from their diseases, so the traducers of the science assert, owe their cure to good fortune rather than to medical skill. Even I do not exclude the operations of fortune, but I think that those who receive bad attention usually have bad luck, and those who have good attention good luck. Secondly, what else but medical skill can be responsible for the cures of patients when they have received medical attention? Such, not content to wait on the shadowy form of Fortune, entrusted themselves to the science of medicine. While the share of chance is excluded, that of science is not. They submitted themselves to its ordinances and they had faith in it; they

considered its apparent nature and the result proved to them its effectiveness.

5. My opponents will say that many sick men have never seen a doctor and yet have recovered from their illnesses. I do not doubt it. But it seems to me that even those who do not employ a doctor may chance upon some remedy without knowing the right and wrong of it. Should they be successful, it is because they have employed the same remedy as a doctor would use. And this is a considerable demonstration of the reality and the greatness of the science, when it be realized that even those who do not believe in it are nevertheless saved by it. For when those who employ no doctors fall sick and then recover, they must know that their cure is due either to doing something or to not doing it. It may be fasting or eating a great deal, drinking largely or taking little fluid, bathing or not bathing, exercise or rest, sleep or wakefulness, or perhaps it is a mixture of several of these that is responsible for their cure. If they benefit, they cannot help but know what benefited them; if they are harmed, what harmed them; but everyone cannot tell what is going to bring benefit or harm beforehand. If a sick man comes to praise or to blame the remedies by which he is cured, he is employing the science of medicine. The failure of remedies too is no less a proof of the reality of the science. Remedies are beneficial only through correct applications, but they are harmful when applied wrongly. Where there are procedures which can be right or wrong, a consideration of these must constitute a science. I assert that there is no science where there is neither a right way nor a wrong way, but science consists in the discrimination between different procedures.

6. If the science of medicine and the profession were concerned in their cures only with the administration of drugs, purges and their opposites, my argument were a weak one. But the most renowned physicians are to be seen employing as therapeutic measures, diets and other ordinances which not even an untaught layman, much less a doctor, could deny were part of their science. There is nothing done which is useless by good doctors, nor is there anything useless in the science of

medicine. The majority of plants and preparations contain substances of a remedial or pharmaceutical nature and no one who is cured without the services of a doctor can ascribe his cure to chance. Indeed, upon examination, the reality of chance disappears. Every phenomenon will be found to have some cause, and if it has a cause, chance can be no more than an empty name. The science of medicine is seen to be real both in the causes of the various phenomena which occur and in the provisions which it takes to meet them, nor will it ever cease to be so.

7. This will suffice as a reply to those who, to the disparagement of medicine, attribute their health to luck. But those who use the example of patients who die from their illnesses as an argument against the efficacy of medicine make me wonder what trustworthy reason leads them to absolve a patient's weakness of character, and impute instead a lack of intelligence on the part of his physician. As if doctors can prescribe the wrong remedies but patients can never disobey their orders! It is far more likely that the sick are unable to carry out the instructions than that the doctors prescribe the wrong remedies. Physicians come to a case in full health of body and mind. They compare the present symptoms of the patient with similar cases they have seen in the past, so that they can say how cures were effected then. But consider the view of the patients. They do not know what they are suffering from, nor why they are suffering from it, nor what will succeed their present symptoms. Nor have they experience of the course of similar cases. Their present pains are increased by fears for the future. They are full of disease and starved of nourishment; they prefer an immediate alleviation of pain to a remedy that will return them to health. Although they have no wish to die, they have not the courage to be patient. Such is their condition when they receive the physician's orders. Which then is more likely? That they will carry out the doctor's orders or do something else? Is it not more likely that they will disobey their doctors rather than that the doctors, whose attitude I have outlined above, will prescribe the wrong remedies? There can be no doubt that the patients are likely to

be unable to obey and, by their disobedience, bring about their own deaths. So they are wrong who attribute the blame to the innocent and exculpate the guilty.

8. There are some too who condemn the science of medicine because doctors are unwilling to tackle incurable cases. They allege that such diseases as the physicians do attempt to treat would get better of themselves in any case, while those that need medical attention are neglected. If medicine were really a science, they say, all should be cured alike. In truth, this arrangement would be a better one if they blamed the doctors for neglecting to treat such madmen as themselves. A man who thinks that a science can perform what is outside its province, or that nature can accomplish unnatural things, is guilty of ignorance more akin to madness than to lack of learning. Our practice is limited by the instruments made available by Nature or by Art. When a man is attacked by a disease more powerful than the instruments of medicine, it must not be expected that medicine should prove victorious. For example, fire is the most powerful caustic known to medicine, although there are many other caustics employed which are less powerful. Now it is not reasonable to call a disease incurable because it does not yield to the weaker remedies, but if it does not respond to the most powerful measures, it is clearly incurable. When fire fails to produce some particular effect, is it not plain that such an effect can only be accomplished by some science other than that whose instrument fire is? The same argument holds good for the failure of other methods employed in medical practice. For these reasons, then, I assert that when the physicians fail, it is the power of the disease which is responsible and not deficiencies in the science of medicine. These critics, then, would have us spend as much time on incurable patients as on those we can do something for. Thus do they impress doctors who are physicians in name alone while they are a laughing-stock to the genuine practitioners of the science. Experts in their professions require neither praise nor blame from such fools as they. Rather do they want criticism from men who have considered what are the full services medicine can

render, what deficiencies remain and, if there are deficiencies, how much must be attributed to the failure of the physicians and how much to the patient.

9. The defence of the other sciences must await another time and another book. Here I am concerned only with the science of medicine, to discuss its nature and how its practice should be judged. I have already demonstrated this in part; I now proceed to the rest. Those who are reasonably proficient in the science of medicine can distinguish two classes of disease. There is a small group in which the signs are readily seen by the eye, those in which the flesh is changed in appearance or in which swellings are demonstrable. Then there is a large group not so easily diagnosed. In the former group, signs can be elicited by sight and touch, for instance, whether the skin be firm or clammy, hot or cold, and each of such signs is of significance. In this group of diseases cure should be complete, not because such diseases are necessarily more amenable to treatment, but simply because the cure has been discovered. And the discoveries were made by no chance comers, but by experts who were in a position to make them. However, anyone can be trained to be an expert who is lacking neither in education nor intelligence.

10. There should be no difficulty, then, in the management of these obvious or external diseases, but the less obvious or internal diseases should not be wholly beyond the power of the science. In this latter group I include disease of the bones and of the cavities of the body. The body contains many hollow organs; there are two which receive and pass on the food and many others which those who have studied them will know. Every part of the body which is covered with flesh or muscle contains a cavity. Every separate organ, whether covered by skin or muscle, is hollow, and in health is filled with life-giving spirit; in sickness it is pervaded by unhealthy humours. The arms, for example, possess such a cavity, as also do the thighs and legs. Even those parts which are relatively poorly covered with flesh contain such cavities. Thus the trunk is hollow and contains the liver, the skull contains the brain and the thorax the lungs. Thus the divisions

of the body may be likened to a series of vessels, each containing within it various organs, some of which are harmful and some beneficial to their possessor. There are in addition many blood vessels and nerves which do not lie loose among the muscles but are attached to the bones and ligaments which form the joints. The joints themselves, in which the ends of the bones turn, are enclosed by capsules which contain a frothy fluid. Should the joint be opened, large quantities of fluid escape and much damage is done.

11. Since these diseases cannot be diagnosed by sight, I call them 'internal diseases' and such is the term employed by the profession. These internal diseases have not been mastered, but they have been mastered as far as possible for the present. The future depends on how far the intelligence of the patients permits the drawing of conclusions and how far the abilities of future investigators are fitted for the task. If the nature of a disease cannot be perceived by the eye, its diagnosis will involve more trouble and certainly more time than if it can. What escapes our vision we must grasp by mental sight, and the physician, being unable to see the nature of the disease nor to be told of it, must have recourse to reasoning from the symptoms with which he is presented. Then when sick men suffer from delay in diagnosis, it is due rather to the nature of the disease and of the patient than to the failure of the physician. It is made more difficult by the fact that the symptoms which patients with internal diseases describe to their physicians are based on guesses about a possible cause rather than knowledge about it. If they knew what caused their sickness they would know how to prevent it. To know the cause of a disease and to understand the use of the various methods by which disease may be prevented amounts to the same thing in effect as being able to cure the malady. When the physician cannot make an exact diagnosis from the patient's description of his symptoms, the doctor must employ other methods for his guidance and any delay in diagnosis is due to the nature of the human frame rather than to a failure of the science of medicine. Medicine aims to cure that which is perceived, treatment being based on judgement rather than on ill-

considered opinion, on energy rather than indifference. The nature of the body is such that a sickness which is clearly seen can be cured. However, a disease may progress rapidly while the diagnosis is slowly becoming apparent to the physician and the patient cannot be saved in time. The progress of a disease is never faster than the speed with which it may be cured and, so long as the administration of remedies begins with the onset of the malady, recovery may be expected. But when the disease has a start because it lurks unseen within the body, a sufferer seeks treatment not when first attacked but only after his malady has gained a firm hold.

12. Thus the efficacy of the science is better demonstrated when it succeeds in relieving an internal malady than if the cure of an apparently hopeless case should be attempted. Different principles guide other crafts. A trade in which the use of fire is necessary cannot be practised in the absence of this element. Further, other crafts are exercised on materials in which mistakes can easily be rectified, as is the case with those which employ wood or hides, or in the craft of engraving on bronze, iron or similar metal. A mistake made in the manufacture of articles from such materials is easily corrected, but the craft cannot be practised at all if one of the materials be missing. Again, the time factor is not of importance and careful workmanship produces better results than speed, although the latter may prove more profitable.[1]

13. But although neither deep abscesses nor diseases of the kidneys nor of the liver nor of other organs situated within the body are visible to the eye, which is the most satisfactory way of observation, medicine has none the less found out means by which a diagnosis may be reached. Such means consist of observations on the quality of the voice, whether it be clear or hoarse, on the respiratory rate, whether it be quickened or slowed, and on the constitution of the various fluids which flow from the orifices of the body, taking into account their smell and colour, as well as their thinness or viscosity. By weighing up the significance of these various signs it is possible to deduce of what disease they are the result, what

---

[1] It is possible that something has been lost from the text of this section.

has happened in the past and to prognosticate the future course of the malady. Even when nature herself does not produce such signs, they may be revealed by certain harmless measures known to those practised in the science. Thus the physicians may determine what remedies should be applied. For instance, a patient may be made to rid himself of phlegm by the administration of certain acid draughts and foods. Thus a visible sign is produced of some underlying disease which could not otherwise be demonstrated to the sight. If a patient be made to walk uphill or to run, abnormalities in respiration will be observed which would not be apparent at rest. By producing sweating in the manner just mentioned the signs of fever can be observed, just as the steam from hot water indicates fire. Substances can be given which, excreted in the urine, or through the skin, reveal the disease better. Then draughts and substances taken by mouth have been discovered, which producing more heat than the cause of some fever, act on that cause and make the fever flow away, a result which would not happen but for the exhibition of such treatment. But both the methods to be employed and the signs produced differ from case to case. As a result the signs may be difficult for the physician to interpret and then cures are slow and mistrust in the power of the doctor persists.

13. That the science of medicine makes use of principles which can be of real assistance has been shown in this work. But it would not be fair to expect medicine to attempt cures that are all but impossible, nor to be unfailing in its remedies. That medicine can be of value is further demonstrated by the skill of those proficient practitioners whose actions are better proof than their words. It is not that such physicians look down on writers, but they believe that most men are more ready to believe what they see than what they hear.

AIRS, WATERS, PLACES

*An essay on the influence of climate, water supply and situation on
health.*

1. Whoever would study medicine aright must learn of the
following subjects. First he must consider the effect of each
of the seasons of the year and the differences between them.
Secondly he must study the warm and the cold winds, both
those which are common to every country and those peculiar
to a particular locality. Lastly, the effect of water on the health
must not be forgotten. Just as it varies in taste and in quality,
so does its effect on the body vary as well. When, therefore, a
physician comes to a district previously unknown to him, he
should consider both its situation and its aspect to the winds.
The effect of any town upon the health of its population varies
according as it faces north or south, east or west. This is of
the greatest importance. Similarly, the nature of the water
supply must be considered; is it marshy and soft, hard as it is
when it flows from high and rocky ground, or salty with a
hardness which is permanent? Then think of the soil, whether
it be bare and waterless or thickly covered with vegetation and
well-watered; whether in a hollow and enervating, or exposed
and cold. Lastly consider the life of the inhabitants themselves; are they heavy drinkers and eaters and consequently
unable to stand fatigue or, being fond of work and exercise,
eat wisely but drink sparely?

2. Each of these subjects must be studied. A physician who
understands them well, or at least as well as he can, could not
fail to observe what diseases are important in a given locality
as well as the nature of the inhabitants in general, when he first
comes into a district which was unfamiliar to him. Thus he
would not be at a loss to treat the diseases to which the inhabitants are liable, nor would he make mistakes as he would
certainly do had he not thought about these things beforehand.
With the passage of time and the change of the seasons, he

would know what epidemics to expect, both in the summer
and in the winter, and what particular disadvantages threatened
an individual who changed his mode of life. Being familiar
with the progress of the seasons and the dates of rising and
setting of the stars, he could foretell the progress of the year.
Thus he would know what changes to expect in the weather
and, not only would he enjoy good health himself for the most
part, but he will be very successful in the practice of medicine.
If it should be thought that this is more the business of the
meteorologist, then learn that astronomy plays a very important part in medicine since the changes of the seasons produce
changes in the mechanism of the body.

3. I shall explain clearly the way in which each of these
subjects should be considered. Let us suppose we are dealing
with a district which is sheltered from northerly winds but
exposed to the warm ones, those, that is, which blow from
the quarter between south-east and south-west, and that these
are the prevailing winds. Water will be plentiful but it will
consist chiefly of brackish surface water, warm in the summer
and cold in the winter. The inhabitants of such a place will
thus have moist heads full of phlegm, and this, flowing down
from the head, is likely to disturb their inner organs. Their
constitution will usually be flabby and they tolerate neither
food nor drink well. It is a general rule that men with weak
heads are not great drinkers because they are particularly liable
to hangovers.

The local diseases are these. The women are sickly and
liable to vaginal discharges; many of them are sterile, not by
nature, but as the result of disease. Miscarriages are common.
Children are liable to convulsions and asthma which are
regarded as divine visitations and the disease itself as 'sacred'.
The men suffer from diarrhoea, dysentery, ague and, in the
winter especially, from prolonged fevers. They are also
subject to pustular diseases of the skin which are particularly
painful at night and also from haemorrhoids. Pleurisy,
pneumonia and other acute diseases are rare since such diseases
do not flourish in a watery constitution. Moist ophthalmia
is not uncommon, but it is neither serious nor of long

duration unless an epidemic breaks out owing to some great change in the weather. Catarrh of the head makes those over fifty liable to hemiplegia. They suddenly become 'sun-struck' or cold. Such then are the diseases of the country, except that changes in the weather may produce epidemics in addition.

4. Let us now take the case of a district with the opposite situation, one sheltered from the south but with cold prevailing winds from the quarter between north-west and north-east. The water supply is hard and cold and usually brackish. The inhabitants will therefore be sturdy and lean, tend to constipation, their bowels being intractable, but their chests will move easily. They will be more troubled with bile than with phlegm; they will have hard heads but suffer frequently from abscesses. The special diseases of the locality will be pleurisy and the acute diseases. This is always the case when bellies are hard. Because of this, too, and because they are sinewy, abscesses commonly appear on the slightest pretext. This is also due to their dryness and the coldness of the water. Such men eat with good appetites but they drink little; one cannot both eat and drink a great deal at the same time. Ophthalmia occurs and is of long duration tending to become both serious and chronic, and the eyes suppurate at an early stage. Those under thirty suffer from epistaxis which is serious in summer. Cases of the 'sacred disease' are few but grave. These men live longer than those I described before. Ulcers do not suppurate nor do they spread wildly. Characters are fierce rather than tame. These then are the diseases to which the men of such a district are liable; others only if some change in the weather provokes an epidemic.

The women suffer largely from barrenness owing to the nature of the water; this is hard, permanently so, and cold. Menstruation, too, does not occur satisfactorily but the periods are small and painful. They give birth with difficulty but, nevertheless, miscarriages are rare. After parturition they are unable to feed their babies because the flow of milk is dried up by the intractable hardness of the water. As a result of difficult labour, abscesses and convulsions commonly occur and wasting disease follows. The children suffer from dropsy of the testicles while they are young, but this disappears as they grow up. Puberty is attained late in such a district.

5. So much for the influence of the warm and cold winds. Let us now consider districts which are exposed to winds from the quarter between north-east and south-east, and then those from the west. Those that face east are likely to be healthier than those facing north or south even if such places are only a furlong apart. These districts do not experience such extremes of heat and cold. The water, to the easterly side, must necessarily be clean, sweet-smelling, soft and pleasant. This is because the early morning sunshine distils dew from the morning mist. The inhabitants are generally of good and healthy complexion unless they are subject to disease. They have loud and clear voices and if, as is probable, local conditions generally are better, they are of better temperament and intelligence than those exposed to the north. The climate in such a district may be compared with the spring in that there are no extremes of heat and cold. As a consequence, diseases in such a district are few and not severe. In general, it may be said that they resemble districts of southern aspect except that the women are prolific and give birth easily.

6. Towns that face west and are thus sheltered from easterly winds while the warm winds and those from the south pass them by, must necessarily have a most unhealthy situation. First, the water is not clear. This is because the air holds the early morning mist and such air, mixing with water, takes away its sparkle, for it does not get the sun on it until late in the day. In summer damp breezes blow and cause dew to fall in the early morning, but for the rest of the day the sun, as it declines, burns up the inhabitants. This tends to make them of poor complexion and sickly and they suffer from all the diseases previously mentioned without exception. Their voices are thick and somewhat hoarse on account of the air which tends to be impure and unhealthy. Not even the northerly gales reach such districts to dispel these characteristics. All the winds that blow are from the west and therefore very wet. The weather of such a district can be compared with the

autumn when there is so great a difference between morning and evening.

7. So much then for the effects, both good and ill, of the various winds. Now I should like to explain what is the effect of different kinds of water, to indicate which are healthy and which unhealthy, and what effects, both good and bad, they may be expected to produce. Water plays a most important part in health. Stagnant water from marshes and lakes will necessarily be warm, thick and of an unpleasant smell in summer. Because such water is still and fed by rains, it is evaporated by the hot sun. Thus it is coloured, harmful and bilious-looking. In winter it will be cold, icy and muddied by melting snow and ice. This makes it productive of phlegm and hoarseness. Those who drink it also have large and firm spleens while their bellies are hard, warm and thin. Their shoulders, the parts about the clavicles and their faces are thin too because their spleens dissolve their flesh. Such men have a great appetite for food and drink. Their viscera will be very dry and warm and thus require the stronger drugs. Their spleens remain enlarged summer and winter and, in addition, cases of dropsy are frequent and fatal to a high degree. The reason for this is the occurrence, during the summer, of much dysentery and diarrhoea together with prolonged quartan fevers. Such diseases, when they are of long standing, cause dropsy in people of this type and this proves fatal. These, then, are the summer ailments. In winter, the younger men are liable to pneumonia and to madness. The older men suffer from a fever called *causus* on account of the dryness of their bellies, the women from tumours and leucorrhoea. The latter are weak in the belly and give birth with difficulty. The foetus is large and swollen. During lactation, wasting and pains occur and menstruation does not become properly re-established. The children are specially liable to rupture and the men to varicose veins and ulcers of the legs. People of such nature cannot be long lived and they become prematurely aged. Moreover, sometimes the women appear to have conceived but, when the time of birth approaches, the contents of the belly disappear. This happens when the womb suffers

from dropsy. Water which produces these things, I consider harmful in every respect.

We now come to the consideration of water from rock springs. It is hard; either from the soil containing hot waters, or from iron, copper, silver, gold, alum, bitumen or nitre. All these substances are formed by the influence of heat. The water from such ground is bad since it is hard, heating in its effect and causes constipation and dysuria.

The best water comes from high ground and hills covered with earth. This is sweet and clean and, when taken with wine, but little wine is needed to make a palatable drink. Moreover, it is cool in summer and warm in winter because it comes from very deep springs. I particularly recommend water which flows towards the east, and even more that which flows towards the north-east, since it is very sparkling, sweet-smelling and light. Water that is salty, hard and cannot be softened, is not always good to drink. But there are some constitutions and some diseases which benefit by drinking such water and these I shall proceed to detail. The best type of this water is that which comes from springs facing the east. The second best from springs facing the quarter between north-east and north-west, especially the more easterly, and the third from springs between north-west and south-west. The worst is the southern variety, the springs facing between south-west and south-east. These water supplies are worse when the winds are southerly than when they are northerly.

Waters should be used in the following way. A man who is in good and robust health need not distinguish between them, but he may drink whatever is to hand at the moment. But if a sick man wishes to drink what is best for him, he would best regain his health by observing the following rule. If his stomach is hard and liable to become inflamed, the sweetest, lightest and most sparkling water is best for him; but if his stomach is soft, moist and full of phlegm, the hardest and saltiest are best since these will best dry it up. The water that is best for cooking and softest is likely to relax and soften the stomach. Hard water that is not softened by boiling tends to make the stomach contract and dries it up. Owing to ignorance, there is a general fallacy about brackish water. Salty water is thought to be a laxative; actually the opposite is the case and permanently hard water tends to make the bowels costive.

8. We now pass from spring water to a consideration of rain water and water from snow. Rain water is very sweet, very light and also very fine and sparkling, since the sun, drawing it up, naturally seizes upon the finest and lightest water, as is proved by the salt which is left behind. The brine is left on account of its thickness and heaviness and becomes salt, but the sun draws up the finest elements because of their lightness. It draws it up not only from ponds, but also from the sea and in fact from any source which contains moisture; and there is nothing that does not contain some. Even from human beings, it draws off the finest and lightest part of the body's humours. A very good proof of this is seen when a man goes and sits in the sun wearing a cloak. Where sunlight falls on the body, no sweat will be seen, but the part which is shaded or protected by something becomes damp with sweat. This is because the sun draws up the sweat and makes away with it; but where the body is shaded, the sweat remains because the sunlight cannot get at it. If the man goes in the shade, the whole body sweats alike because the sun is no longer on him. Rain water, being composed of a mixture of so many elements, quickly becomes rotten on standing and exhales a foul smell. But when it has been drawn up into the air, it travels round and mixes with the air; the dark and cloudy part is separated and becomes cloud and mist, while the clearest and lightest part is left, sweetened by the sun heating and boiling it. Everything is sweetened by boiling. So long as it is scattered and does not mass together, it remains floating in the air. But when it is gathered and collected suddenly by the assault of contrary winds, then it falls wherever there happens to be the densest cloud. This is most likely to happen when a wind has gathered some clouds together and is driving them along and then another wind suddenly confronts it with another mass of clouds. Then the first cloud is stopped and the following ones pile up on it till it becomes thick and black and

dense, and its weight causes it to turn to rain and fall. Rain water, therefore, is likely to be the best of all water, but it needs to be boiled and purified. If not, it has a foul smell and causes hoarseness and deepness of the voice in those that drink it.

Water from snow and ice is always harmful because, once it has been frozen, it never regains its previous quality. The light, sweet and sparkling part of it is separated and vanishes leaving only the muddiest and heaviest part. You may prove this, if you wish, by measuring some water into a jar and then leaving it out in the open air on a winter's night in the coldest spot you can find. Next morning bring it back into the warmth again and, when it has thawed, measure it a second time. You will find the quantity considerably less. This shows that in the process of freezing, the lightest and finest part has been dried up and lost, for the heaviest and densest part could not disappear thus. For this reason I consider such water to be the most harmful for all purposes.

9. The effect of drinking water collected from many different sources, that is, from large rivers fed by smaller streams and from lakes into which many streams flow from different directions, is to cause a propensity to stone, gravel in the kidneys, strangury, pain in the loins and rupture. The same is true of water brought long distances from its source. The reason for this is that no two sorts of water can be alike but some will be sweet, some salt and astringent and some from warm springs. When they are all mixed they quarrel with one another and the strongest is always the dominant. But each one has not always the same strength and sometimes one is dominant, sometimes another according to which wind is blowing. One will be made strong by the north wind, another by the south and so on. Such water will leave a sediment of sand and slime at the bottom of the jar and it is by drinking this that the diseases mentioned above are caused. There are, however, certain exceptions and these I shall detail.

Those whose stomachs are healthy and regular, and whose bladders are not subject to inflammation, nor in whom the neck of the bladder is overmuch obstructed, pass water easily

H

and nothing collects in the bladder. But if the belly is liable to fever the same must be true of the bladder, and when this organ is heated with fever, the neck of the bladder becomes inflamed and does not allow the urine to pass which instead becomes heated and condensed. The finest and clearest part is separated, passes through and is voided. The densest and cloudiest part is gathered together and precipitates in small pieces at first and then in larger ones. The gravel formed is rolled round by the urine and coalesces to form a stone. When water is passed this falls over the neck of the bladder, and being pressed down by the pressure of the urine, prevents the urine from being passed. Great pain is thus caused. As a result, children suffering from stone rub or pull at their private parts because they think that in them lies the cause why they cannot make water. The fact that people who suffer from stone have very clear urine is proof that the densest and muddiest part remains in the bladder and collects there. This is the explanation of most cases of this disease but, in children, stones may also be caused by milk. If milk is not healthy but too warm and bilious-looking, it heats the stomach and the bladder and the urine is heated and a similar result is produced to that already described. Indeed, I assert that it is better to give children wine watered down as much as possible for this neither burns the veins nor dries them up too much. Female children are less liable to stone because the urethra is short and wide and the urine is passed easily. Neither do they masturbate as the males do, nor touch the urethra. In the female the urethra is short; in males it is not straight and it is narrow as well. Moreover, girls drink more than boys.

10. Now let us consider the seasons and the way we can predict whether it is going to be a healthy or an unhealthy year. It is most likely to be healthy if the signs observed at the rising and the setting of the stars occur normally, when there is rain in the autumn, when the winter is moderate being neither too mild nor excessively cold, and when rain falls seasonably in spring and in summer. But if the winter be dry with northerly winds prevailing and the spring wet with southerly winds, the summer will of necessity be feverish and productive

of ophthalmia and dysentery. For when stifling heat succeeds while the ground is still wet from the spring rains and southerly winds, the heat will be twice as great. Firstly because of the soaked warm earth and secondly because of the blazing sun; and, moreover, men's stomachs will not be toughened nor the brain firm. In such a spring the flesh cannot but become flabby and this predisposes to acute fevers, especially in those of phlegmatic constitution. Dysentery is likely to attack women and those of watery diathesis. Should the etesian winds blow and there is bad weather and rain at the rising of the Dog Star, then it may be hoped that these bad conditions will come to an end and that the autumn will be a healthy one. But if there is no amelioration in the conditions there is a danger of fatalities among women and children; the elderly are in the least danger. Those who recover are liable to quartan fevers in which dropsy may supervene.

If the winter is wet and mild with southerly winds and this is followed by a wintry dry spring with the wind in the north, the effect will be as follows. First, women who happen to be pregnant and approaching term in the spring are likely to have miscarriages. Or, if they do give birth, the babies are so weak and sickly that either they die at once or, if they survive, they are frail and weak and very liable to disease. The men are liable to dysentery and dry ophthalmia, while some will suffer from catarrh of the head which may spread to the lungs. It is those who are full of phlegm, as well as the women, who are likely to suffer from dysentery since the phlegm flows down from the brain on account of their moist constitutions. On the other hand, those who are full of bile suffer from dry ophthalmia on account of the warmth and dryness of the flesh, while the old, owing to the permeability and exhaustion of the blood vessels, suffer from catarrh. This last illness may prove suddenly fatal to some, while others are afflicted with a right- or left-sided hemiplegia. The explanation of these diseases is this. When the winter is warm with wet south winds neither the brain nor the blood vessels become consolidated. Thus, when spring comes with dry cold northerly winds, the brain becomes stiff and cold just when it ought to thaw and become purified by running of the nose and hoarseness. It is the sudden change when the heat of summer comes that is responsible for these diseases.

Districts which are well situated with regard to the sun and the winds and which have a good water supply are the least affected by such changes in the weather; those badly situated with regard to the sun and the winds and which draw their water from marsh or lake, the most. If the summer be dry, diseases are short lived, but if it is wet they last long and there is the danger of a sore appearing on the slightest pretext if the skin be broken. Diarrhoea and dropsy occur towards the termination of illnesses under such conditions because the tissues are not dried up.

If the summer is rainy with southerly winds and the autumn similar, the winter will necessarily be unhealthy. Those of phlegmatic constitution and those over forty years old may suffer from *causus*, while those who are full of bile suffer from pleurisy and pneumonia. If the summer is dry with northerly winds and the autumn wet with the wind in the south, the winter brings a danger of headache and gangrene of the brain. Further, there is likely to be hoarseness, running at the nose and cough and, in some cases, consumption. If the autumn is rainless with northerly winds and there is rain neither under the Dog Star nor at Arcturus, this weather suits best those who are naturally phlegmatic and of a watery constitution and also women. But it is most inimical to those of a bilious disposition because they become dried up too much. This produces dry ophthalmia and sharp fevers which last a long time and also, in some cases, 'black bile' or melancholy. The reason for this is found in the drying up of the more fluid part of the bile while the denser and more bitter part is left behind. The same is true of the blood. But these changes are beneficial to those of phlegmatic habit so that they become dried up and start the winter braced up instead of relaxed.

11. Anyone making observations and drawing deductions on these lines can foretell most of the effects which follow changes in the weather. It is particularly necessary to take precautions against great changes and it is inadvisable to give

a purge, to cauterize or to cut any part of the belly until at least ten days have passed after such a change. The most dangerous times are the two solstices, especially midsummer, and the equinoxes. Both of these latter times are considered dangerous but more especially the autumnal one. Care must also be taken at the rising of certain stars, particularly the Dog Star and Arcturus. Similarly, discretion must be exercised at the setting of the Pleiads. It is at such times that the crisis is reached in the course of diseases; some prove fatal and some are cured, but all show some kind of change and enter a new phase.

12. I now want to show how different in all respects are Asia and Europe, and why races are dissimilar, showing individual physical characteristics. It would take too long to discuss this subject in its entirety but I will take what seem to me to be the most important points of difference.

Asia differs very much from Europe in the nature of everything that grows there, vegetable or human. Everything grows much bigger and finer in Asia, and the nature of the land is tamer, while the character of the inhabitants is milder and less passionate. The reason for this is the equable blending of the climate for it lies in the midst of the sunrise facing the dawn. It is thus removed from extremes of heat and cold. Luxuriance and ease of cultivation are to be found most often when there are no violent extremes, but when a temperate climate prevails. All parts of Asia are not alike, but that which is centrally placed between the hot and the cold parts is the most fertile and well wooded; it has the best weather and the best water, both rain water and water from springs. It is not too much burnt up by the heat nor dessicated by parching drought; it is neither racked by cold nor drenched by frequent rains from the south or by snow. Crops are likely to be large, both those which are from seed and those which the earth produces of her own accord. But as the fruits of the latter are eaten by man, they have cultivated them by transplanting. The cattle raised there are most likely to do well, being most prolific and best at rearing their young. Likewise, the men are well made, large and with good physique. They differ little among themselves in size and physical development. Such a land resembles the spring time in its character and the mildness of the climate.

.   .   .   .

16.[1] So much for the differences of constitution between the inhabitants of Asia and of Europe. The small variations of climate to which the Asiatics are subject, extremes both of heat and cold being avoided, account for their mental flabbiness and cowardice as well. They are less warlike than Europeans and tamer of spirit, for they are not subject to those physical changes and the mental stimulation which sharpen tempers and induce recklessness and hot-headedness. Instead they live under unvarying conditions. Where there are always changes, men's minds are roused so that they cannot stagnate. Such things appear to me to be the cause for the feebleness of the Asiatic race, but a contributory cause lies in their customs; for the greater part is under monarchical rule. When men do not govern themselves and are not their own masters they do not worry so much about warlike exercises as about not appearing warlike, for they do not run the same risks. The subjects of a monarchy are compelled to fight and to suffer and die for their masters, far from their wives, their children and friends. Deeds of prowess and valour redound to the advantage and advancement of their masters, while their own reward is danger and death. Moreover, such men lose their high-spiritedness through unfamiliarity with war and through sloth, so that even if a man be born brave and of stout heart, his character is ruined by this form of government. A good proof of this is that the most warlike men in Asia, whether Greeks or barbarians, are those who are not subject races but rule themselves and labour on their own behalf. Running risks only for themselves, they reap for themselves the rewards of bravery or the penalties of cowardice. You will also find that the Asiatics differ greatly among themselves, some being better and some worse. This follows from the variations of climate to which they are subject, as I explained before.

.   .   .   .

[1] At this point some paragraphs have been lost, and the order of what remains is uncertain.

13. Such then is my opinion of Egypt and Libya. I will now discuss the area to the east-north-east as far as Lake Maeotis,[1] for this is the boundary between Europe and Asia. The people inhabiting these regions differ more among themselves than those discussed previously on account of the changeability of the weather and the nature of the terrain. And what is true of the soil is true of the men. Where the weather shows the greatest and the most frequent variations, there the land is wildest and most uneven. You will find mountains, forests, plains and meadows. But where there is not much difference in the weather throughout the year, the ground will be all very level. Reflection will show that this is true of the inhabitants too. Some men's characters resemble well-wooded and watered mountains, others a thin and waterless soil, others plains or dry bare earth. Climates differ and cause differences in character; the greater the variations in climate, so much the greater will be differences in character.

14. I will leave out the minor distinctions of the various races and confine myself to the major differences in character and custom which obtain among them. First the Macrocephali; no other race has heads like theirs. The chief cause of the length of their heads was at first found to be in their customs, but nowadays nature collaborates with tradition and they consider those with the longest heads the most nobly born. The custom was to mould the head of the newly-born children with their hands and to force it to increase in length by the application of bandages and other devices which destroy the spherical shape of the head and produce elongation instead. The characteristic was thus acquired at first by artificial means, but, as time passed, it became an inherited characteristic and the practice was no longer necessary. The seed comes from all parts of the body, healthy from the healthy parts and sickly from the sickly. If therefore bald parents usually have bald children, grey-eyed parents grey-eyed children, if squinting parents have squinting children, why should not long-headed parents have long-headed children? The custom of binding

[1] The Sea of Azov.

the head has also become obsolete through intercourse with other peoples.

15. I pass now to consider the people who live near the river Phasis[1]. Their land is marshy, warm, wet and thickly covered with vegetation. Violent rainstorms occur there frequently at all seasons of the year and the inhabitants live in the marshes. Their houses are built on the water of wood and reeds and they do very little walking to go to town or to market, but sail up and down along the many canals in dug-out canoes. They drink warm stagnant water which has been rotted by the sun and swollen by the rains, and the Phasis itself is the most sluggish and stagnant of all rivers. The crops that grow there are all poor, feeble and do not ripen well owing to the superabundance of water which interferes with the ripening process. The ground is often covered with mist. As a result of this the Phasians have peculiar constitutions. They are big and stout and their joints and veins are obscured by flesh. Their skin is yellowish as if they had jaundice and their voices, because they breathe the air which is moist and damp and not clean, are the deepest known. They have little stamina but become quickly tired. The climate varies very little and the prevailing winds are southerly, except for one local breeze which sometimes blows a stiff warm gale. They call this wind the Kenkhron. The north wind never blows hard even when it does blow.

17[2]. In Europe, on the other hand, and living round Lake Maeotis, there is a special race of Scythians which differs from all other peoples. They go by the name of Sauromatae. Their women ride horses and shoot arrows and hurl javelins from the saddle and they fight in campaigns as long as they remain virgins. Nor do they lose their virginity until they have killed three of their enemies and have offered such sacrifices as are prescribed by ritual law. But once a woman has taken to herself a husband she does not ride again unless military necessity should require their total forces to take to the field. The women have no right breast since their mothers heat a specially made iron and apply it to the breast while they are

---

[1] Rion.   [2] See note on page 102.

still children. This prevents the breast from growing and all the strength and size of it goes into the right arm and shoulder instead.

18. As regards the appearances of other tribes of Scythians, the same is true of them as is true of the Egyptians, namely, that they have certain racial characteristics, but differ little among themselves. They differ, however, from the Egyptians in that their peculiarities are due to cold instead of to heat. The so-called Scythian desert is a grassy plain devoid of trees and moderately watered, for there are large rivers there which drain the water from the plains. Here live the Scythians who are called nomads because they do not live in houses but in wagons. The lighter wagons have four wheels but some have six, and they are fenced about with felt. They are built like houses, some with two divisions and some with three, and they are proof against rain, snow and wind. The wagons are drawn by two or three yokes of hornless oxen; hornless because of the cold. The women live in these wagons while the men ride on horseback, and they are followed by what herds they have, oxen and horses. They stay in the same place as long as there is enough grass for the animals but as soon as it fails they move to fresh ground. They eat boiled meat and drink the milk of mares from which they also make a cheese.

19. So much then for their mode of life and customs. As regards their physical peculiarities and the climate of their lands, the Scythian race is as far removed from the rest of mankind as can be imagined and, like the Egyptians, they are all similar to one another. They are the least prolific of all peoples and the country contains very few wild animals and what there are are very small. The reason for this is their situation in the far north under the Rhipaean mountains from which the north wind blows. The sun shines most brightly towards its setting in the summer and then it warms them only for a very short time and not very much. In addition, the winds from warm lands do not reach as far, as a rule, or, if they do, they are weak. Instead, northerly winds, chilled with snow and ice and charged with great rains, blow continuously

and never leave the mountains which makes them most inhospitable. During the daytime mist often covers the plains where the people live and, in fact, winter is nearly continuous all the year round. The summer lasts only a few days and these are not very summery for the plains are highly situated, bare of trees and are not engirdled by mountains, but slope from the north. The only wild animals found there are those small enough to shelter underground. The cold weather together with the barrenness of the ground, which affords neither warmth nor shelter, prevents their growth. There are no great nor violent changes with the seasons, the climate remaining very much the same all the year round. The people differ little in physique as they always eat similar food, wear the same clothes winter and summer, breathe moist thick air, drink water from snow and ice and do no hard work. The body cannot become hardened where there are such small variations in climate; the mind, too, becomes sluggish. For these reasons their bodies are heavy and fleshy, their joints are covered, they are watery and relaxed. The cavities of their bodies are extremely moist, especially the belly, since, in a country of such a nature and under such climatic conditions, the bowels cannot be dry. All the men are fat and hairless and likewise all the women, and the two sexes resemble one another. Owing to the lack of variation in the weather, there is no interference with the coagulation of the semen unless there is some inter-current disease.

20. As a proof of this moistness of the constitution, I may instance the following. You will find that the majority of the Scythians, especially those who are nomads, are cauterized on the shoulders, arms, wrists, chests, hips and loins. This is done simply for the softness and moistness of their constitutions because otherwise they could neither bend their bows nor put any weight into throwing the javelin. But when they have been cauterized the moisture is dried out of their joints and their bodies become more sinewy and stronger and their joints may then be seen. They grow up flabby and stout for two reasons. First because they are not wrapped in swaddling clothes, as in Egypt, nor are they accustomed to horse-riding

as children which makes for a good figure. Secondly, they sit about too much. The male children, until they are old enough to ride, spend most of their time sitting in the wagons and they walk very little since they are so often changing their place of residence. The girls get amazingly flabby and podgy. The Scythians have ruddy complexions on account of the cold, for the sun does not burn fiercely there. But the cold causes their fair skins to be burnt and reddened.

21. People of such constitution cannot be prolific. The men lack sexual desire because they are so flabby and because of the softness and coldness of their bellies, a condition which least inclines men to intercourse. Moreover, being perpetually worn out with riding they are weak in the sexual act when they do have intercourse. These reasons suffice as far as the men are concerned. In the case of the women, fatness and flabbiness are also to blame. The womb is unable to receive the semen and they menstruate infrequently and little. The opening of the womb is sealed by fat and does not permit insemination. The women, being fat, are easily tired and their bellies are cold and soft. Under such conditions it is impossible for the Scythians to be a prolific race. As a good proof of the sort of physical characteristics which are favourable to conception, consider the case of serving wenches. No sooner do they have intercourse with a man than they become pregnant, on account of their sturdy physique and their leanness of flesh.

22. Further, the rich Scythians become eunuchs and perform women's tasks on an equal footing with them and talk in the same way. Such men they call Anarieis. The Scythians themselves attribute this to a divine visitation and hold such men in awe and reverence, because they fear for themselves. Indeed, I myself hold that this and all other diseases are equally of divine origin and none more divine nor more earthly than another. Each disease has a natural cause and nothing happens without a natural cause. My own explanation of this disability of the Scythians is this. As a result of horse-riding they are afflicted with varicosity of the veins because their feet are always hanging down from their mounts. This is followed by lameness and, in severe cases, those affected drag

their hips. They treat themselves by their own remedy which is to cut the vein which runs behind each ear. The haemorrhage which follows causes weakness and sleep and after this some, but not all, awake cured. My own opinion is that such treatment is destructive of the semen owing to the existence of vessels behind the ears which, if cut, cause impotence and, it seems to me that these are the vessels they divide. Consequently when they come into the presence of their wives and find themselves impotent, they do not perhaps worry about it at first, but when after the second and third and more attempts the same thing happens, they conclude that they have sinned against the divinity whom they hold responsible for these things. They then accept their unmanliness and dress as women, act as women and join with women in their toil.

That it is the rich Scythians, those of the noblest blood and the greatest wealth, and not their inferiors, who suffer from this disease is due to horse-riding. The poor suffer less because they do not ride. Yet, surely, if this disease is more to be considered a divine visitation than any other, it ought to affect not only the rich but everyone equally. Rather, the poor should be specially liable to it if the gods really do delight in honours and the admiration of men and bestow favours in return. It is the rich who make frequent sacrifice and dedication to the gods because they have the means. The poor, being less well provided with goods, sacrifice less and accompany their prayers with complaint. Surely it is the poor and not the rich who should be punished for such sins. Really, of course, this disease is no more of 'divine' origin than any other. All diseases have a natural origin and this peculiar malady of the Scythians is no exception. The same thing happens in other races. Those who ride the most suffer most from varicose veins, pain in the hips and gout and they are the less able to perform their sexual functions. This is the fate of the Scythians. They are the most effeminate race of all mankind for the reasons I have given; and because they always wear trousers and spend so much of their time on horseback so that they do not handle their private parts, and, through cold and exhaustion, never have even the desire for sexual intercourse. Thus they have no sexual impulses in the period before they lose their virility.

23. The remaining peoples of Europe differ widely among themselves both in size and appearance owing to the great and frequent climatic changes to which they are subject. Hot summers and hard winters, heavy rains followed by long periods of drought, all these occasion variations of every kind. It is reasonable that these changes should affect reproduction by variations in the coagulability of the semen so that its nature is different in summer and winter, in rainy weather and times of drought. I believe this to be the reason for the greater variation among individuals of the European races, even among the inhabitants of a single city, than is seen among Asiatics and also why they vary so much in size. When the weather changes often, abnormalities in the coagulation of the semen are more frequent than when the weather is constant. A variable climate produces a nature which is coupled with a fierce, hot-headed and discordant temperament, for frequent fears cause a fierce attitude of mind whereas quietness and calm dull the wits. Indeed, this is the reason why the inhabitants of Europe are more courageous than those of Asia. Conditions which change little lead to easy-going ways; variations to distress of body and mind. Calm and an easy-going way of living increases cowardice; distress and pain increase courage. That is one reason for the more warlike nature of Europeans. But another cause lies in their customs. They are not subjects of a monarchy as the Asiatics are and, as I have said before, men who are ruled by princes are the most cowardly. Their souls are enslaved and they are unwilling to risk their own lives for another's aggrandisement. On the other hand, those who govern themselves will willingly take risks because they do it for themselves. They are eager and willing to face even the worst of fates when theirs are the rewards of victory. It is clear, then, that the tradition of rule has no small influence on the courage of a people.

24. In general it may be said that these are the differences between Europe and Asia. There exist in Europe, then, people differing among themselves in size, appearance and courage,

and the factors controlling those differences are those I have described. Let me summarize this plainly. When a race lives in a rough mountainous country, bare of trees, and well watered, where great differences of climate accompany the various seasons, there the people will be of large physique, well-accustomed to hardihood and bravery, and with no small degree of fierceness and wildness in their character. On the other hand, in low-lying, stifling lands, full of meadows and where the water is warm, the people will be neither large nor slight, but rather broad in build, fleshy and black-haired. Their complexions are dark rather than fair and they are phlegmatic rather than bilious. Bravery and hardihood are not an integral part of their natural characters although these traits can be created by training. The people of a country where rivers drain the surface water and rain water have clear complexions and good health. But where there are no rivers and the drinking water is taken from lakes or marshes, the people will necessarily be more pot-bellied and splenetic. People who live in countries which are high, level, windswept and rainy tend to be of large stature and to show little variation among themselves. They are also of a less courageous and less wild disposition. In countries where there is a light waterless soil devoid of trees and where the seasons occasion but small changes in climate, the people usually have hard sinewy bodies, they are fair rather than dark and they are strong-willed and headstrong in temperament. Places where changes of weather are most frequent and of the greatest degree show the greatest individual differences in physique, temperament and disposition among the inhabitants.

The chief controlling factors, then, are the variability of the weather, the type of country and the sort of water which is drunk. You will find, as a general rule, that the constitutions and the habits of a people follow the nature of the land where they live. Where the soil is rich, soft and well-watered and where surface water is drunk, which is warm in summer and cold in winter, and where the seasons are favourable, you will find the people fleshy, their joints obscured, and their tissues watery. Such people are incapable of great effort. In addition, such a people are, for the most part, cowards. They are easy-going and sleepy, clumsy craftsmen and never keen or delicate. But if the land is bare, waterless and rough, swept by the winter gales and burnt by the summer sun, you will find there a people hard and spare, their joints showing, sinewy and hairy. They are by nature keen and fond of work, they are wakeful, headstrong and self-willed and inclined to fierceness rather than tame. They are keener at their crafts, more intelligent and better warriors. Other living things in such a land show a similar nature. These, then, are the most radically opposed types of character and physique. If you draw your deductions according to these principles, you will not go wrong.

PROGNOSIS

The importance of being able to foretell the course of an illness, and an account of the significance of various signs.

1. It seems to be highly desirable that a physician should pay much attention to prognosis. If he is able to tell his patients when he visits them not only about their past and present symptoms, but also to tell them what is going to happen, as well as to fill in the details they have omitted, he will increase his reputation as a medical practitioner and people will have no qualms in putting themselves under his care. Moreover, he will the better be able to effect a cure if he can foretell, from the present symptoms, the future course of the disease.

It is impossible to cure all patients; that would be an achievement surpassing in difficulty even the forecasting of future developments. But seeing that men die before the physician is able to bring his skill to grapple with the case—some owing to the violence of the disease die before they have summoned the doctor, some as soon as he arrives; some live one day, others a little longer—in view of this, an understanding of such diseases is needed. One must know to what extent they exceed the strength of the body and one must have a thorough acquaintance with their future course. In this way one may become a good physician and justly win high fame. In the case of patients who were going to survive, he would be able to safeguard them the better from complications by having a longer time to take precautions. By realizing and announcing beforehand which patients were going to die, he would absolve himself from any blame.

2. The signs to watch for in acute diseases are as follows. First study the patient's *facies*; whether it has a healthy look and in particular whether it be exactly as it normally is. If the patient's normal appearance is preserved, this is best; just as the more abnormal it is, the worse it is. The latter appear-

ance may be described thus: the nose sharp, the eyes sunken, the temples fallen in, the ears cold and drawn in and their lobes distorted, the skin of the face hard, stretched and dry, and the colour of the face pale or dusky. Now if at the beginning of an illness the face be such and one's judgement lacks confirmation from other signs, the patient should be asked whether he has suffered from insomnia, from severe diarrhoea, or if he has ravening hunger. If he admits to any of these things, the case must be judged less severe than if it were otherwise, for where the facial appearance is due to any of these causes a crisis will be reached in a day and a night. But if he admits none of these things, and if there is no improvement within the prescribed time, it must be realized that this sign portends death.

Should the illness have passed the third day before the face assumes this appearance, the same questions as I mentioned before should be asked, and an examination of the whole body made for other signs, paying particular attention to the eyes. For if they avoid the glare of light, or lacrimate without due cause, or squint, or the one becomes smaller than the other, or ecchymoses occur in the whites of the eyes, or if the whites are livid or show the presence of tiny dark veins, or if bleariness appear around the eyes, or if the eyes wander, or project, or are deeply sunken, or if the whole complexion of the face be altered; then all these things must be considered bad signs and indicative of death.

The appearance of the eyes in sleep should also be noted, for if some of the white shows when the eyes are closed, so long as it is not due to diarrhoea, the taking of drugs, or the normal habit in sleep, it is a bad sign and especially fatal. If the eyelid becomes swollen or livid, or likewise the lip or the nose, together with one of the other signs, it may be known that death is at hand. It is also a fatal sign if the lips are parted and hang loose and become cold and white.

3. When the physician visits the patient, he should find him lying on one side or the other, with his hands, neck and legs slightly bent, and with the whole body lying relaxed. For this is how most healthy people lie. The best manner of lying in

I

bed is that which most nearly resembles the manner of healthy people. It is not so good if the patient lies on his back with his hands and legs extended; while if he should have fallen forwards away from the bed towards his feet, that is worse still.

If he should be found with his feet uncovered, unless they are exceptionally warm, and with his hands and legs flung about at random, it is a bad sign because it is evidence of restlessness.

It is a fatal sign to sleep with the mouth continuously wide open, and if the patient lies on his back with his legs very much bent and intertwined. It is also bad if a patient sleeps on his stomach unless this is his normal habit when well; such a posture indicates delirium or abdominal pain.

For the patient to want to sit up when the disease is at its height is a bad sign in all acute diseases, but worst of all in cases of pneumonia. For a patient with fever to grind his teeth, unless this be a habit continued from childhood, is a sign of madness and death. If this occurs during delirium, it is a sign that the disease has already taken a fatal turn.

Inquiries should be made about any sore which has been discovered to ascertain whether it existed prior to the illness, or whether it has developed during the course of the illness. For, if the patient is about to die, before death the sore will become either livid and dry or pale and hard.

4. The following points about the gestures of the hands should be noted. In cases of acute fever or of pneumonia and in brain-fever and headache, it is a bad sign and portends death if any of the following things are noted: if the hands are waved in front of the face, or make grabs at the air, or pull the nap off cloth, or pull off bits of wool, or tear pieces of straw out of the wall.

5. Rapid breathing indicates either distress or inflammation in the supra-diaphragmatic organs. Deep breaths taken at long intervals are a sign of delirium. If the expired air from the mouth and nostrils is cold, death is close at hand. Regular respiration is to be considered a most important indication of recovery in all the acute diseases which are accompanied by fever and reach the crisis within forty days.

6. Fits of sweating are excellent in all acute diseases when

they occur on the critical days, and mark the final end of the fever. They are also good when the whole body is involved, and show that the patient is taking the disease more easily. But those which conform to neither of these circumstances are of no advantage. The worst kinds of sweating are those which are cold and occur only round the head and neck; these, if accompanied by a high fever, mean death; if by a milder fever, a long illness.

7. The most satisfactory condition of the hypochondrium is when it is painless, but is soft and smooth on both sides. On the other hand, precautions must be taken if it is inflamed and painful, or taut, or if there is a difference in level between the two sides. Should there also be a throbbing in the hypochondrium, it is a sign of violent disturbance or delirium. In such cases, the appearance of the eyes should be noted; if the eyes move rapidly, it is highly probable that the patient is mad.

A hard and painful swelling of the hypochondrium which involves the whole of that area is a very bad sign. If it be only on one side, it is less fraught with danger if it is on the left side. When such swellings are present at the beginning of an illness, it is an indication of the danger of a speedy death; but if the patient lasts more than twenty days while remaining febrile and without the swelling subsiding, then it will suppurate. In these cases, a violent epistaxis occurs during the first period and this is very helpful, but the patient should be asked whether he has a headache, or if his sight is dim. If either of these symptoms were present, it would incline to provoke the epistaxis. Epistaxis is more likely to occur in patients under the age of thirty-five.

Swellings which are soft, painless and pit on pressure with the finger, cause delayed crises but are less to be feared than the former kind. But if the patient continue febrile for more than sixty days without the swelling subsiding, then an empyema is being formed. The same is also true of swellings in the belly.

In brief, then, painful hard large swellings mean danger of a speedy death; soft, painless swellings which pit on pressure, mean protracted illness.

Swellings in the belly are less likely to be productive of abscess than those in the hypochondria, and those below the navel are the least likely to suppurate. Epistaxis is particularly to be expected in association with swellings in the upper parts. Whenever a swelling lasts a long time, the formation of an empyema at that site must be expected.

When suppuration occurs, the following points should be noted. Of those which point externally, the best sort are those which are small, bulge outwards as much as possible and come to a sharp head. The worst sort are those which are large and flat, and which do not come to anything like a sharp head. Of those which burst internally, the best are those which have no connection with the exterior, and which are localized, painless and show a uniform colouring all over the external surface. The best sort of pus is that which is white, smooth, homogeneous and least foul-smelling. That of the opposite sort is the worst.

8. All cases of dropsy arising from acute diseases are bad. For, besides not getting rid of the fever, they are particularly painful and liable to cause death. In most cases dropsy starts from the flanks and the loins, but sometimes from the liver. In those cases where the dropsy starts from the flanks and loins, the feet swell and long-lasting diarrhoea occurs which neither puts an end to the pain in the flanks and loins nor empties the belly.

9. It is a bad sign if the head, hands and feet are cold while the belly and sides are warm. It is best that the body should be warm all over and equally soft.

The patient should turn over easily and be light when lifted up. If he should appear rather heavy, in the hands and feet as well as in the rest of the body, there is greater danger. If, in addition to this heaviness, the nails and fingers become livid, death is immediately to be expected. But if the fingers or the feet become completely black, this is less fatal than if they are livid. Nevertheless, other signs should be taken into consideration as well, for if the patient appears to be bearing up well under the disease, or if he displays in addition to this any of the signs which betoken recovery, it is probable that the disease will result in abscess formation with survival of the patient, although those parts will be lost which have turned black.

Drawing up of the testicles or private parts indicates distress or death.

10. As regards sleep, the patient should follow our natural habit and spend the day awake and the night asleep. If this habit be disturbed, it is not so good. Nevertheless, it is better that he should sleep during the morning and early afternoon than later. It is worst of all when he sleeps neither night nor day; it may be that pain and distress is keeping him awake, or this sign of insomnia may precede delirium.

11. It is best when the stools are soft and formed, and passed at the hour customary to the patient when in health; their bulk should be proportionate to the amount of food taken. Such stools indicate a healthy condition of the lower bowel. But if the stools be fluid, it is best that they should not be accompanied by a noise, nor passed in small quantities at frequent intervals; the continual getting up is exhausting for the patient and prevents him from sleeping. If he should pass large stools frequently, there is a risk of his fainting. He should, according to how much he eats, pass stools two or three times during the day and once during the night. The larger stool should be passed in the morning as he was accustomed. The stools should become more solid towards the crisis when the disease is being cured. They should be light brown and not too foul-smelling. It sometimes happens that round worms are passed with the stools toward the crisis when the disease is being cured.

In every illness, the belly should be loose and the stools of good size. It is a bad sign if the stools are very watery, or white, or particularly yellowish or frothy. It is also bad if they are small, sticky, white, yellowish and smooth. Signs more indicative of death are when they are dark, or livid, or oily, or rust-coloured and foul-smelling. Variety in the stools denotes a longer illness, but is no less a sign of a fatal outcome. Such stools are those which are full of shreds, bloody, bilious, green and dark stools; sometimes such constituents are passed together, sometimes separately.

It is best to emit wind without a noise or breaking wind; but it is better to emit it even with a noise than to repress or smother it. All the same, wind emitted in this manner indicates that there is something wrong internally, or that the patient is delirious, if, at least, the emission of wind is involuntary.

Pains and swellings in the hypochondria, if they are fresh and not accompanied by inflammation, are dispersed by a rumbling gathering of wind in the hypochondrium, especially if it be passed through the body and voided with the stools and urine. It may be passed through by itself. It is also a good thing if the gathering of wind moves down to the lower regions.

12. Urine is best when there is a white, smooth, even deposit in it the whole time up to the crisis of the disease, for this indicates recovery and a short illness. If there should be intervals when clear urine is passed, and the white, smooth, even deposit appears only at times, this means that the illness will be prolonged and that recovery is less certain. If the urine should be pink with a pink smooth sediment, although such indicates an illness even longer than in the previous case, it is a certain sign of recovery. Sediment like barley-meal in the urine is bad, and it is even worse if the sediment resembles flakes. Thin white sediment is a very bad sign, and it is even worse if it resembles bran. Clouds suspended in the urine constitute a good sign if they are white, a bad one if they are dark.

So long as the urine is thin and yellowish-red, the disease is not ripened. If the illness is prolonged and the urine remain of that colour, there is a danger that the patient may not last out till ripening occurs. Urine which is foul-smelling or watery or dark or thick is more a sign of death. In the case of men and women, dark urine is worst; in the case of children, watery urine.

When a patient continues to pass thin raw urine for a long time and the other signs indicate recovery, the formation of an abscess should be expected in the parts below the diaphragm.

When grease forms patterns like cobwebs on the surface of the urine, this constitutes a warning, for it is a sign of wasting.

When urine contains clouds, it should be noted whether they are towards the top or the bottom, and what is their colour. Those which sink and have the colours previously mentioned as favourable are to be judged a good sign. Those which rise and have the colour said to be unfavourable constitute a bad sign. You must not be deceived if these appearances result merely from a diseased condition of the bladder, for they may then indicate not a disease of the whole body, but merely of that organ.

13. The most helpful kind of vomiting is that in which the matter brought up consists of phlegm and bile, as well-mixed as possible, and is neither thick nor particularly great in quantity. If it is not well-mixed, it is less good. The vomiting of dark green, livid or dark, no matter which of these colours, must be considered a bad sign. If the same patient should vomit material of all these colours, his condition is already fatal. The quickest death is denoted by the vomiting of livid matter if it has a foul smell. All rotten and foul odours coming from vomited material are bad.

14. In all diseases which affect the lungs and sides, sputum should be brought up early and, in appearance, the yellow matter should be thoroughly mixed with the sputum. It is not so good if it only comes about some while after the beginning of the pain, that the sputum is brought up and it is yellow, or light brown, or the cause of much coughing, or if it be not thoroughly mixed. It is a sign of danger if the yellow matter is not diluted; and white, sticky and nummular sputum is not beneficial. It is worse if it should be a marked pale green and frothy. If it should be so undiluted as to appear dark, this is even worse still. It is also bad if the lungs are not cleared and nothing is produced, but the throat remains full of bubbling matter.

In all diseases of the lungs, running at the nose and sneezing is bad, whether it existed before the illness or supervened during its course. But in other diseases which are likely to prove fatal, sneezing is beneficial. In cases of pneumonia, the production at the beginning of the illness of yellow sputum mixed with a little blood is a good indication of recovery. But when this occurs on or after the seventh day, it is less certainly good. All sputa are bad which do not relieve the pain; the worst are those which are dark in colour as stated above. The production of any sputum which relieves pain is rather better.

15. When aches arising in these regions are not relieved by the production of sputum or evacuation of the bowels, or by venesection or the administration of drugs and special regimens, you must know that an empyema is present. Those empyemas which begin to suppurate while the sputum is still bilious are especially signs of a fatal issue, whether the bilious matter is brought up separately from the pus or together with it.

Most specially, if the empyema appears to start from sputum of this sort when the disease is in its seventh day, the patient who brings up such sputum may be expected to die on the fourteenth day, unless a good sign makes its appearance. The good signs which may appear are these: to bear the illness easily, to have good respiration, to be free from pain, to cough up sputum easily, to have the body evenly warm and soft all over, not to suffer from thirst, to have the urine, stools, sleep and sweating of the types described above as good. If all these signs appear the patient is not likely to die; but if only some of these signs appear, he may die although he will live longer than fourteen days. The opposites of these are bad signs; to bear the illness hardly, to draw deep and frequent breaths, to suffer continued pain, to have difficulty in coughing up sputum, to have violent thirst, to have the body unevenly warm with the abdomen and sides very warm and the forehead, hands and feet cold, to have the urine, stools, sleep and sweating of the types described above as bad. If any of these signs appear subsequent to the bringing up of sputum of this description, the patient may die in less than fourteen days, either on the ninth or eleventh. This is the inference which should be drawn from observing this kind of sputum; it is particularly likely to indicate death and may not give the patient his fourteen days.

The most reliable forecast is that which takes into account the good and the bad signs which appear in addition. Other

empyemata burst as a rule, some on the twentieth day, some
on the fortieth and some reach sixty days.

16. The beginning of an empyema may be reckoned for
calculation from the day on which the patient first had a fever,
or when he had a rigor, or when he said that a heaviness
replaced the pain in the spot where he feels discomfort. These
things occur at the start of an empyema. The discharge of pus
must be expected according to the stated intervals reckoned
from this day.

In cases where the empyema is unilateral, the patient should
be made to turn over on the side affected and then asked
whether he has an ache in that side. Or, if one side be hotter
than the other, he should be made to lie on the healthy side
and then be asked if he feels as if a weight were hanging on
him from above. If such is the case, the empyema is on whichever side the heaviness is felt.

17. All empyemata may be recognized by the following
signs. First of all, the fever does not intermit, but remitting a
little during the day, becomes more acute at night. Many fits
of sweating occur. A desire to cough is aroused, but nothing
is brought up to speak of. The eyes become sunken, and the
cheeks are flushed. The finger-nails become curved and the
fingers become warm, especially at their tips. Swellings which
come and go are observed in the feet. Blisters form on the
body and the patients show no desire for food.

Chronic empyemata show these signs and considerable
reliance may be placed in them. Those which will not last
long are indicated by their showing the sort of signs which
appear at the start of the empyema, and also by the patient
suffering somewhat from difficulty with breathing. Whether
it will burst sooner or later may be determined from the
following signs—if pain occurs at the beginning, and dyspnoea,
cough and expectoration continue, bursting may be expected
in twenty days or even less. If the pain be less acute and the
other signs are normal, bursting may be expected after twenty
days. Pain, dyspnoea and expectoration must always precede
the evacuation of pus.

Patients with empyema who are most likely to survive are

those whom the fever leaves on the same day as the abscess bursts, and who quickly regain their appetite, lose their thirst and who pass small firm stools, and from whom white smooth pus, all of the same colour without inflammation, flows out and is cleared away without pain or coughing. These are the best signs and patients who show them speedily recover, and failing these, the best signs are their nearest approximations.

Those patients die when the fever does not leave them on the same day as the abscess bursts, but in whom, after an apparent departure, it reappears and gives them a high fever. They suffer from thirst and anorexia and diarrhoea, and the pus is greenish-yellow and livid, or phlegmatic and frothy. When all these signs appear, death is certain; when some appear, but not all, the patient may die or he may recover after a prolonged illness. But indications should be drawn not only from the special signs concerned with the empyema itself, but also from all the other signs as well.

18. When abscess formation from pneumonic conditions occurs near the ears and suppurates downwards with the production of a fistula, the patient recovers.

Some complications must be suspected under the following conditions: if the fever is continuous and the pain incessant, if the sputum does not appear normal, and if the stools are neither bilious nor loose and homogeneous, if the urine is not thick and containing much sediment. In such cases, if the other signs of recovery are favourable, the formation of abscesses can be expected. These sometimes occur in the lower regions, in cases where some of the inflammation is located near the hypochondrium; sometimes in the upper regions where the hypochondrium remains soft and painless. In such cases, the patient having for some time suffered from dyspnoea, regains normal respiration without any apparent cause.

Abscess formation in the legs is always beneficial in severe and critical cases of pneumonia, but most specially so when it follows a change in the nature of the sputum. For if the swelling and pain comes on when the sputum has become purulent instead of yellow and when it is being expectorated, this constitutes the surest sign that the patient is going to recover and that the abscess will quickly become painless and resolve. But if the sputum is not expectorated well and urine with a satisfactory sediment does not appear, there is a danger that the limb may become lame or give a good deal of trouble.

If the abscess disappears without any expectoration of sputum while the fever continues, it is a bad sign for there is a danger that the patient may become delirious and die.

It is the older people who are more likely to die when empyemata complicate pneumonia, whereas in the case of empyema from other causes, death is more frequent among younger people.

19. When pain accompanied by fever attacks the loins and lower regions, they are specially fatal if the pain leaves the lower regions and fastens on the diaphragm. Attention should therefore be paid to the other signs. If another bad sign appears as well, the case is hopeless. But if other bad signs do not appear when the pain leaps up to the diaphragm, there is a good chance of an empyema forming.

It is always a bad sign if the bladder becomes hard and painful; most fatal if this is accompanied by continuous fever. The distress occasioned by the bladder alone is enough to kill the patient, while the bowels remain unopened under such circumstances except for the forcible passage of hard matter. The passage of urine resembling pus with a white smooth sediment terminates the condition. If there is no improvement in the urine and the bladder does not become soft, and if the fever is continuous, the patient is likely to die early in the disease. This condition occurs most frequently in children between the ages of seven and fifteen.

20. Fevers reach their crises in the same number of days whether the patient survives or dies. The mildest fevers, and those which give the surest indications of recovery, cease on or before the fourth day. Those which are the most severe and accompanied by the worst signs cause death on the fourth day or earlier. The first bout of a fever ends in this period, the second later until the seventh day, the third till the eleventh day, the fourth till the fourteenth day, the fifth till the seven-

teenth day, the sixth till the twentieth day. In the case of most acute diseases, the bouts continue for twenty days, each bout adding four days at a time. But none of these periods can be computed in whole numbers exactly; neither the solar year nor the lunar month are of such a length as to be counted in whole numbers of days.

Subsequently, addition continues in the same way so that the first period contains thirty-four days, the second forty days and the third sixty days. It is very difficult to distinguish at the beginning between those fevers which are going to reach a crisis in a long period for they are very much alike in the way they start. However, the possibility should be borne in mind from the first day and reconsidered every time a period of four days is added and then the way in which the disease is developing will not escape you. Quartan fevers too follow the same pattern.

Those fevers which are going to reach the crisis in a short time are easier to recognize, for they show considerable differences from the start.

The patients who are going to recover have good respiration and no pain, they sleep at night and display other signs of recovery. Those who are going to die have dyspnoea, insomnia and delirium, and display other very bad signs. Thus, once this is recognized, calculations must be made which are based on the period and the appropriate additions as the disease moves towards its crisis. The crises which women undergo after child-birth follow the same plan too.

21. Severe continuous headache accompanied by fever is a certain sign of death if any of the other fatal signs occur as well. If there are no such signs, but the headache lasts more than twenty days while the fever continues, an epistaxis or some other abscession to the lower regions should be expected. An epistaxis or empyema may also be expected while the headache is still young, especially if it is temporal or frontal. Epistaxis is more likely with patients under thirty-five; empyema with older men.

22. Acute earache accompanied by continuous and severe fever is a bad sign; there is a danger that the patient may

become delirious and die. In view of the dangerous nature of this condition, special attention must be paid from the first day to any other signs. Younger men die on the seventh day or sooner from this malady; older men much more slowly for they are less liable to fever and delirium and for this reason their ears suppurate before they reach a fatal stage. Nevertheless, at such ages, relapse is usually fatal. The younger men die before the ear suppurates. When white pus flows from the ear, there is a chance that a young man may recover if some other good sign appears as well.

23. Pharyngeal ulceration accompanied by fever is a bad sign and, if any other sign of those previously mentioned as bad appears as well, it may be said in advance that the patient is in danger. The worst kind of sore throat, and that which carries off those who suffer from them most quickly, is that which shows no obvious sign either in the throat or in the neck, but produces excessive pain and orthopnoea. Suffocation occurs on the first, second, third or fourth day. Those cases which are in other respects very similar and suffer pain, but in which the throat swells up and becomes inflamed, are also very fatal but the disease is more protracted than the previous sort.

When both the throat and the neck are inflamed, these sore throats last longer. Those suffering from them recover especially if a rash appears on the neck and chest and the erysipelas does not turn inwards. If the erysipelas does not disappear in the critical number of days, or if an external swelling does not appear, or if pus is not coughed up easily and without distress, this constitutes a sign of death or of a relapse of the inflammation. It is safest when the erysipelas turns outwards as much as possible; if it turns towards the lungs, it causes delirium and empyema usually follows.[1]

24. A relapse is to be expected in those cases where a fever departs either without any sign of resolution appearing or if it departs on days other than the critical ones. Whenever a fever is prolonged while the patient appears likely to recover and suffers no pain by reason of any inflammation or any other apparent cause, an abscession accompanied by swelling and

---

[1] A short passage which seems to be an interpolation is omitted here.

pain into one of the joints, most probably one of the lower ones, should be expected. Such abscessions occur particularly and in a shorter time in patients under the age of thirty years.

The formation of an abscession should be suspected at once if the fever lasts more than twenty days without remission. This is less likely to happen with older people in whom the fever lasts longer. If the fever is continued, such an abscession should be expected, but if it intermits and attacks in an irregular fashion and continues thus till autumn is at hand, it is likely to develop quartan periodicity. Just as people under thirty are specially liable to abscession, so those above that age are specially liable to quartan fevers.

It should be observed that during the winter abscessions are more likely and take longer to depart, but they are less liable to return.

When a patient with a fever which is unlikely to cause death professes a headache and a blackness before the eyes, or if heartburn accompany this, bilious vomiting will occur. If a rigor occurs as well, and the parts below the diaphragm are cold, vomiting will occur even sooner. If the patient takes any food or drink at this time, it will very quickly be brought up again. When such distress begins on the first day, the greatest distress will be on the fourth and fifth days; recovery will be about the seventh. In most cases, however, distress begins on the third day and the disease reaches its height on the fifth, departing on the ninth day or on the eleventh. When the distress begins on the fifth day, and in other respects the condition is similar to that previously described, the crisis occurs on the fourteenth day. These symptoms are specially common in tertian fevers in the case of adults. Younger people do suffer from them in tertians too, but more often in more continued fevers and genuine tertians.

When in this kind of fever the patient complains of headache, but instead of darkness before the eyes his sight becomes dim or is dazzled, and instead of heartburn there is contraction of the hypochondrium on one side or the other unaccompanied by either pain or inflammation, epistaxis is more likely to occur than vomiting. Even so, epistaxis is more probable in the young; those over thirty are less liable to it, but more liable to vomiting.

Children are likely to have convulsions if the fever is high and if they are constipated, if they are wakeful, frightened, cry and change colour, turning pale, livid or red. This most commonly happens in children under the age of seven. As they grow up and reach adult years, they are no longer likely to be attacked by convulsions in the course of a fever, unless one of the most severe and worst signs appears as well, as happens in inflammation of the brain. Whether the children and the others will recover or die must be judged by the whole total of signs as described in each case.

This concludes my remarks on acute diseases and those arising from them.

25. Anyone who is to make a correct forecast of a patient's recovery or death, or of the length of his illness, must be thoroughly acquainted with the signs and form his judgement by estimating their influence one on another, as has been described in speaking of urine, sputa and other subjects. The physician must be quick to think of the trend of any diseases that are epidemic from time to time, and the climatic conditions must not escape him. It should, however, be observed that the indications and signs have invariably the same force, the bad being always bad and the good good, in every year and under all climatic conditions. The truth of those described in this treatise has been proved in Libya, in Delos and in Scythia. It should therefore be realized that there is nothing remarkable in being right in the great majority of cases in the same district, provided the physician knows the signs and can draw the correct conclusions from them. There is no point in seeking the name of any disease which has not been mentioned, for all which reach their crisis in the periods described may be recognized by the same signs.

REGIMEN IN ACUTE DISEASES

The effect of various regimens upon an ailing body. Apparently a polemic treatise written to refute certain doctrines held by the neighbouring school of medicine at Cnidus.

1. The authors of the book called *Opinions from Cnidus* have given a correct account of the symptoms in patients suffering from various diseases and, in some cases, of the ultimate effects of the disease. Thus far indeed anyone might go, if he inquired diligently of each patient what his symptoms were, without being a physician. But these authors have omitted a great deal of what the physician should learn from his patient without his telling him; details which vary from case to case but the interpretation of which may sometimes be of vital importance.

2. Whenever their interpretation of the symptoms leads them to prescribe a cure, my opinions differ from theirs very considerably. Nor is this the only criticism I have to make, for, in addition, they employ too few remedies. Thus, apart from acute diseases, they generally prescribe opening medicine and recommend their patients whey and milk to drink.

3. Of course, if these remedies were satisfactory and were adapted to the diseases for which they were prescribed, I should think very highly of them seeing that so few were sufficient. But this simply is not the case. Later writers, however, have approached the subject in a more scientific way and enumerated the diets to be given to patients in various diseases. But no one so far has written any considerable work on regimen in general, although this is a most important omission. Some of these authors were unaware of the multiplicity of the different ways in which each disease may present itself; thus they made mistakes when they tried to set down clearly the number of individual diseases. It is not easy to count accurately if a different name is given to every morbid condition differing but slightly from another; and unless a disease has the same name in all its forms it will appear to be a different disease.

4. I believe that attention should be paid to all the details of the science (of healing). Measures requiring to be done well and exactly must be performed well and exactly; where speed is essential, with speed; where cleanliness is required, with cleanliness; and where pain is to be avoided, the patient should be treated so as to cause the minimum of pain. All such things should be done considerably better by the physician than by another.

5. I would single out for praise the physician who particularly excels in the treatment of acute diseases, for these cause the greatest number of deaths. By acute diseases are meant the conditions which earlier doctors have named pleurisy, pneumonia, brain-fever and *causus*, and conditions resembling them which usually show continued fever. For in the absence of an epidemic of a disease of the plague type, many more die of these conditions than all the others together.

6. Laymen, far from recognizing those who excel in the treatment of acute diseases, generally praise or blame any cure that is different. A good indication that the common people are at their most unintelligent in discussing these diseases, is that such cases give quacks their reputations as physicians. It is easy enough to learn the names of the things given to treat such patients, and if anyone talks of barley water, or of such and such a wine, or of hydromel, the layman thinks that all doctors, both good and bad, mean exactly the same thing. On the contrary, it is in such matters that their differences are clearly shown.

7. It seems to me worth while recording facts which in spite of their importance are not generally known to the medical profession, and to state what is harmful and what beneficial in the treatment of patients. For instance it is not generally known why some physicians all their lives give their patients gruel which is unstrained, thinking this is the right way to effect a cure; while others regard it as of the highest importance that the patient should not swallow a single grain of barley, as they think this causes great harm, but strain the barley-water through a linen cloth before giving it to their patients. Some again give neither gruel nor barley-water; others give it only

K

during the first seven days of the disease and yet others give it till the crisis be reached.

8. Physicians are quite unaccustomed to propound such questions, and perhaps they do not appreciate them when they are propounded. The science of medicine has fallen so low in popular estimation as not to seem the science of healing at all. As a result, if in the acute diseases at least, practitioners differ so widely that the diet prescribed by one is regarded as bad by another, the science could almost be compared to divination. Seers think the same bird to be of good omen if it appears on the left and bad if it appears on the right, while other seers hold exactly the opposite view; and there are similar contradictions in divination by inspection of an animal's entrails.

9. I assert that this study of regimen is much to be recommended, and it is something closely allied to the most numerous and the most vital studies which compose the science of medicine. To the sick it is a powerful aid to recovery, to the healthy a means of preserving health, to athletes a means of reaching their best form and, in short, the means by which every man may realize his desire.

10. Barley-gruel seems to have been correctly selected as the most suitable cereal to give in these acute diseases and I have a high opinion of those who selected it. Its gluten is smooth, consistent and soothing; and is slippery and fairly soft; it is thirst-quenching and easily got rid of in case this be necessary. It contains nothing to produce constipation or serious rumbling, nor does it swell up in the stomach for during cooking it swells up to its maximum bulk.

11. Patients who take gruel in these diseases should not, as a general rule, fast on any day. They should take it without interruption unless the use of a purge or an enema renders a break necessary. Those who are accustomed to two meals a day should be given gruel twice daily; those who are accustomed to take only one meal a day should take gruel once only on the first day and thereafter it is permissible to increase this gradually and to give it twice a day if there seems to be any need for it. At the beginning of an illness it should be given

sparingly, nor should it be very thick; in fact, the patient should take only as much as he requires to allay an empty feeling.

12. If the disease is drier than one would like, the patient should be given a drink of either hydromel or wine—whichever is appropriate and this will be discussed later—before the gruel, and increases in the quantity of gruel should be avoided. But if the mouth is moist and the pulmonary secretions are produced properly, the quantity of gruel should, as a general rule, be increased. For the sooner moist discharges appear and the more pronounced they are, the sooner will the crisis come, whereas delay in their appearance means that the crisis too will be delayed. Such is the general rule on these particular points.

13. There are many other important signs by which prognosis may be made; they will be passed over now to be treated later. The larger the stools, the more nourishment should be given until the crisis. This is specially so at the crisis and then extra large amounts should be given for the next few days. At least, this regimen should be adopted in those cases in which the crisis appears to take place on the fifth, seventh or ninth day; by so doing, precautions will have been taken for the following even day as well as the odd day of the crisis. Later, gruel should be given at first, giving place to solid food later.

14. This treatment is generally successful if thick gruel is taken from the beginning. In cases of pleurisy, the pain stops spontaneously as soon as the patient begins to bring up any considerable amount of sputum and to be purged. Evacuation of discharges is much more complete and empyema less likely to occur on this regimen than if a different diet were taken. The crisis is more simple, more easily reached and less liable to be followed by a rclapse.

15. The best barley should be used for gruel and it should be cooked as well as possible, especially if you intend to use only the barley-water. Apart from its other excellencies, the slipperiness of gruel makes the barley itself quite safe to swallow, for it does not adhere or lodge anywhere in its passage through the thorax. It is most slippery, thirst-

quenching, easily digested and weakest if it is really well cooked; all of which qualities are desirable.

16. A course of dieting on such gruel may be very harmful unless measures are taken to make it sufficient. Thus, if a patient has food retained in the stomach it will, unless he be made to evacuate some of it before being given gruel, only exacerbate any pain he already has, or give him one if he has none, and it will make respiration more rapid. This is bad because it dries up the lung and causes distress in the hypochondrium, the abdomen and diaphragm. Moreover, no gruel should be given to patients in whom the pain in the side be persistent in spite of warm fomentations, while the sputum is viscid and unripe and retained, unless the pain be relieved by relaxing the bowels or by cutting a vein, whichever may be indicated; if gruel is given to patients in such a condition, they will very quickly die.

17. For these and other similar reasons those who take thick gruel die within a week; in some cases after partly going out of their minds, in others choked by orthopnoea and stertorous breathing. It used to be thought that such patients had been the subject of a stroke, particularly because when they died the side was livid like a bruise. The reason for this appearance is that they die before the pain is allayed, for difficulty in breathing quickly sets in. Because the sputum becomes viscid and unripened, expiration is impeded causing wheezing in the bronchial tubes and thus, as has already been said, increased frequency of the respiration leads rapidly to asthma. When a patient reaches this condition, his case is generally desperate. The retained sputum actually prevents the intake of breath and forces it quickly to be expelled. Thus one thing is added to another. The retained sputum increases the rate of respiration and this in itself makes the sputum viscid so that it cannot run away. This may happen not only as the result of the untimely taking of gruel, but much more so if the patient eats or drinks anything less suitable.

18. In most respects, the additional precautions to be observed are the same whether the gruel is taken thick or strained to make barley-water. If neither of them, but only

drink is taken, the treatment to be given is sometimes different. The general rules are as follows.

19. If the fever begins soon after the patient has taken a meal and the bowels have not been opened, whether it be accompanied by pain or not, the diet of gruel should be withheld until it is judged that the food has passed to the lower part of the intestines. Fluids should be given and oxymel is recommended if there is pain, hot in winter and cold in summer. If there is acute thirst, hydromel and water may also be taken. If there is pain or any of the dangerous signs appear, but only after the seventh day or if the patient be strong, then gruel should be given. Should there be no evacuation of food previously consumed after recent food has been taken, an enema should be given to patients who are strong and in the prime of life; patients who are too weak should be given a suppository unless the bowels are opened satisfactorily of their own accord.

20. There is one time both at the beginning and, indeed, throughout the illness when gruel should not be given and that is when the feet are cold. It is then specially important not to administer any fluids, as well as to withhold gruel. But when warmth descends to the feet, then it may be given. It must be remembered that this is a time of great importance in all diseases, and not least in acute diseases and those accompanied by fever. Barley-water especially and gruel too should not be given without accurate observation of the signs which have been mentioned.

21. A pain in the side, whether it appears at the beginning of the illness or at a later stage, should first be treated in the ordinary manner in an attempt to remove it by hot fomentations. The best type of fomentation is hot water in a skin or bladder, or in an urn of bronze or earthenware. For comfort, something soft should first be put against the side. It is also good to apply a large soft sponge which has been dipped in hot water and wrung out. The warm object should be protected on top as in this way it stays hot longer and this also prevents steam reaching the patient's nostrils, unless of course this is regarded as beneficial; there are occasions when it is

needed. Barley and vetch may also be used if mixed with a little vinegar, sharper than one would drink, to soften it. It is then heated and sewn up in bags which are applied. Bran may be used in the same way. For dry fomentations, salt or millet is best, baked in woollen bags; millet is light and comforting.

22. Such a softening process also removes aches that extend up to the clavicles. Bleeding is not so efficacious in relieving pain. If the distress is not relieved by hot fomentations, heating should not be long continued as this dries up the lungs and causes empyema. If the pain causes a heavy feeling spreading towards the clavicle or arm, or about the breast or above the diaphragm, the inner vein at the elbow should be cut and you should not be afraid of drawing a large quantity of blood until, instead of running clear and red, it becomes either much redder or turns livid; either of these may happen.

23. If the pain is below the diaphragm and does not seem to extend towards the clavicles, the belly should be softened with either black hellebore or purple spurge, adding to the black hellebore, parsnip, seseli, cummin, anise or some other fragrant herb, and to the purple spurge the juice of silphium. These are also similar in effect if mixed with each other. But black hellebore gives a better evacuation and one more likely to produce a crisis, while purple spurge is better for breaking up wind. Both stop pain as do many other purgatives, but they are the best of those I know. Purgatives administered in the gruel are also helpful, so long as they are not too unpleasant owing to bitterness or any other unpleasant taste, or owing to the size of the dose or colour or anything else that may make them distasteful.

24. When the patient takes the purge, he should immediately be given a quantity of gruel not noticeably less than that to which he is accustomed. It is however customary to give no gruel during the purging. When purging stops, then less gruel than usual should be given, the amount subsequently being increased so long as the pain remains alleviated and no other contrary indication appears.

25. If it is proposed to give only barley-water, my advice is the same. I believe it to be better to start giving gruel right

away than to empty the body and then start a diet of gruel on the third, fourth, fifth, sixth or seventh day, unless the disease has already reached a crisis within that period. In this case too the same preparations should be made as have been described.

26. Such then is my opinion about the administration of gruel. As regards the sort of drink a patient should take, the gist of what I am going to say is very much the same. I know that physicians do the exact opposite of what is correct; they all want to dry up their patients for two or three days or more at the beginning of their illness, and then start to administer gruel and fluids. Perhaps it seems reasonable to them that when a violent change takes place in the body, it should be countered by a change equally violent.

27. A change in regimen may have considerable beneficial effects, but the change must be made in the right way and with intention. It is also important that the diet administered after the change should be correct. Those on a diet of thick gruel would suffer most if the change were incorrectly made, but those who are receiving only drink and those who take only barley-water would also suffer, the latter least.

28. Lessons should be drawn from our experience of what diets are best for men in health. If sudden changes in various diets are found to make a great difference to healthy people, it is only to be expected that they will have a great effect in disease, and the greatest in the acute diseases. It is well known that a low diet of food and drink is on the whole a surer way to health than violent changes from one diet to another. Sudden changes will harm those who take two meals a day and those who take one, and make them ill. Likewise, people who have not made a habit of taking breakfast are at once made ill if they take it. Their body feels heavy and they are weak and sluggish. If on top of this they dine they get heartburn. In some cases, too, loose stools are passed because the belly has been subjected to an unaccustomed load having been used to drying up and not being twice filled and having twice to digest a meal.

29. It is helpful in such cases to compensate for the change. An unwanted breakfast should be followed by a sleep, just as

we go to bed for the night after dinner. In winter, care should be taken to avoid shivering; in summer to avoid being too warm. If sleep will not come, a slow prolonged stroll, with no stops, should be taken. Dinner should be dispensed with, or only a little taken of something which can do no harm. Still less should be drunk and nothing watery. Such a man would suffer still more if he were to eat to repletion three times a day; still more if he did so more often. There are, however, many people who take three good meals a day without any ill effects, if they are accustomed to it.

30. It is also true that those who have been accustomed to eating two meals a day become weak, ill, slack at all kinds of work and suffer from heartburn, if they miss breakfast. Their intestines feel unsupported, they pass warm pale green urine and their stools are dried up. Sometimes, in addition, the mouth becomes bitter, the eyes sunken, the temples throb and the extremities become cold. As a rule those who have had no breakfast are unable to eat any dinner, or if they do their bellies feel heavy and they sleep less soundly than if they had previously breakfasted.

31. Seeing that such things can happen to healthy people as the result of half a day's change in diet, it seems best in sickness not to give more nor less than the patient is accustomed to.

32. If a man, who contrary to his usual habit took only one meal, were to fast all day and eat his usual dinner, it is probable that it would lie still more heavily on him, seeing that he felt ill through missing breakfast and found his dinner lie heavy on him. The longer the fast which was suddenly broken, the more he would suffer.

33. An unaccustomed fast may be compensated for as follows. Excessive cold, heat or fatigue should be avoided, for all these would occasion distress. Less dinner should be taken than is usual and this should consist of the moist rather than dry foods. Drink should not be watery, and should not be less than usual in proportion to what is eaten. The next day a light breakfast should be taken and then a gradual return made to a normal diet.

34. People suffer most from these changes in diet when they

are of bilious disposition. Those who are phlegmatic generally suffer least discomfort from fasting, and so suffer less from taking only one meal a day contrary to their normal habits.

35. This will be sufficient to demonstrate that the most violent changes affecting our natures and constitutions are the most productive of illness. One must not without good reason order severe fasting, nor give food when a disease is at its height and is accompanied by inflammation, nor must one make sudden changes in either direction.

36. Many other related points concerning the belly could be mentioned, to show how well it puts up with food and drink to which it is accustomed, even if this is not naturally good. On the contrary, it has difficulty in digesting food and drink to which it is unaccustomed even if they are not bad in themselves.

37a. It would scarcely appear remarkable if pain in the stomach were caused by taking an excess of meat, or by garlic or silphium, either the juice or the stalk, or anything of that kind. But it is surprising to learn how much distress, trouble, wind and colic in the stomach is caused by eating barley-cakes when one is accustomed to bread; or how much heaviness and constipation bread can cause one accustomed to barley-cakes. It is surprising, too, what thirst and sudden fullness is caused merely by eating bread when it is still warm, owing to its drying nature and the slowness with which it passes. Similarly, differing effects are produced by bread which is over-milled or made of unsifted meal if eaten by one not accustomed to it, or barley-cakes that are too dry or too moist or too sticky. Again, new barley-meal may affect those not accustomed to it, or that which is old, those accustomed to new.

Similarly, a sudden change in habit in which wine is substituted for water as a beverage, or *vice versa*, or the substitution of watered for neat wine: one produces distention of the upper part of the belly and wind in the lower, the other causes throbbing of the veins, heaviness in the head and thirst. Again, a change from white to red wine, even though both are equally strong, can cause an upset. All these things can cause many disturbances in the body. It would therefore appear less remarkable that a sudden change from a sweet to a strong wine, or *vice versa*, should fail to preserve a balanced constitution.

37b. I must however make a small concession here to the opposite school of thought. Such conditions are corrected by reversing the regimen, because changes of diet in these cases are not accompanied by changes in the body. The body is not growing stronger so as to need more food, nor weaker so as to need less.

38. The severity and character of each disease must be considered in relation to the patient and his customary diet both solid and liquid. Any increase is specially to be avoided since it is often advantageous to prescribe a total fast in those cases where the patient appears likely to be able to survive until the disease reaches its height. The cases in which this should be done will be described.

39. Much that is akin to what has been said might be added, but the following is the most convincing evidence. Not only is it related to the subject that forms my main topic, but it is itself a most opportune lesson. Those who are stricken with an acute disease sometimes eat food the very same day as the disease begins, some eat on the next day. Some swallow whatever is to hand, and some even drink *cyceon*.[1] All these possibilities are more harmful than if some other diet had been followed. However, mistakes are much less serious at this stage than they would be if the patient fasted totally for two or three days and then started eating on the fourth or fifth day. It would be still worse if he should fast on these days and then subsequently start to take these things before the disease had passed its height, for it is quite obvious that such a course is generally fatal unless the disease be extremely mild. But mistakes at the beginning are not so serious and are much easier to remedy. This is, I think, a most important lesson: during the first days of an illness the patient must not be forbidden any kind of gruel if gruel or solid food is shortly afterwards to be prescribed.

40. There is in fact utter ignorance among those who take

---

[1] A mixture of wine, cheese and barley.

barley-gruel that it is harmful if they have fasted for two or three days previously, and those who take barley-water are unaware that it too may do them harm unless they start taking it in the right way. It is however known, and the point is carefully observed, that it is very bad for the patient to drink barley-gruel before the disease has reached its height if he has been accustomed to barley-water.

41. All these things constitute clear evidence that physicians mishandle their patients' diets. They prescribe fasting in those diseases in which patients are going to be given gruel and who should not be prepared by fasting. They prescribe a change from fasting to gruel in just those cases in which a change should not be made. For the most part they prescribe the change from fasting to gruel at exactly the stage when it is beneficial to reduce the diet even to a complete fast, that is, when the disease is approaching a paroxysm.

. . . .[1]

43. I observe also that physicians are not acquainted with the way in which one can distinguish the various causes of weakness during the course of an illness; which is due to fasting, which to some other provocation, which to distress and to the violence of the disease, or to distinguish the various states and appearances engendered by the constitution and condition of each one of us. Yet life or death may hang upon the ability to distinguish and to recognize such things.

44. It is in fact a serious fault to give a patient who is weak from distress and the violence of the disease more drink or gruel or solid food under the impression that his weakness is due to fasting. It is also an outrage to fail to realize that a patient's weakness is due to fasting and to make him worse by prescribing abstinence. Not only is this latter mistake dangerous, though less so than the former, but it is more likely to involve the physician in ridicule. For another physician or even a layman has only to come along and, having recognized what has happened to the patient, give him something to eat and drink in defiance of the other's orders, and the error is

---

[1] Section 42, which is clearly an interpolation from another work, is omitted.

plain to all to see. Such are particularly the occasions which expose the practitioner to ridicule since the physician or layman who intervenes seems almost to have raised a man from the dead. The signs by which each condition can be distinguished will therefore be described.

.   .   .   .[1]

45. This however is very similar to conditions in the belly. For if the whole body is rested much more than is usual, there is no immediate increase in strength. In fact, should a long period of inactivity be followed by a sudden return to exercise, there will be an obvious deterioration. The same is true of each separate part of the body. The feet and limbs would suffer in the same way if they were unaccustomed to exercise, or were exercised suddenly after a period of rest. The same is true of the teeth and of the eyes, and in fact of every part of the body. A softer bed than usual or one harder than usual causes distress, and sleeping in the open hardens the body.

46. A single illustration of all this will suffice. Suppose a man has a wound on the lower part of the leg which is neither very serious nor quite trifling, and not the sort which will heal very rapidly or very slowly. If from the first day he has it attended to and takes to his bed and never raises his leg, inflammation is less likely and he will be cured much more quickly than if he should walk about during treatment. If however on the fifth or sixth days, or even later, he should get up and walk about, he will suffer more distress than if he had been walking about from the beginning of the cure. And if at this stage he suddenly exerted himself much, he would suffer much more than if he had followed the other course of treatment and exerted himself to the same extent. All these facts hang together and constitute a proof that any change much in excess of what is moderate is harmful.

47. To take an immoderate amount of food after a long fast does very much more harm to the belly than to fast from a hearty diet, and may be compared with the effect on the other parts of the body of over exertion after a long period of rest.

[1] Something appears to be missing here.

Just as the body should be given a complete rest and idleness, and slackness follow a long period of strenuous effort, so should the belly be given a rest from full feeding as otherwise it will cause pain and distress throughout the body.

48. Most of what I have said relates to changes from one diet to another. This is generally useful information, but something in particular must be added about the change from fasting to the taking of gruel in acute illnesses and this change must be made according to the instructions I give. Moreover, gruel must not be given until the disease has ripened or some sign has appeared either in the intestines, indicating starvation or irritation, or in the hypochondrium. These signs I shall describe.

49. Severe insomnia makes food and drink harder to digest. On the other hand, a change in the other direction relaxes the body and brings languor and headache.

50. The various effects in acute illnesses of the different sorts of wine, sweet or strong, white or red, and of hydromel, water or oxymel, can be judged from the following indications.

Sweet wine is less likely to produce headache than is heavy wine, it has less effect upon the mind and, as regards the internal organs, it is more easily passed than the other but causes enlargement of the spleen and liver. It is most unsuitable for those with bitter bile for it makes them thirsty. It may cause wind in the upper internal organs, but it does not trouble the lower organs in this way. Wind caused by sweet wine does not easily escape but lingers about the hypochondrium. It is also, generally speaking, less easy to pass in the urine than is strong white wine. Sweet wine produces more sputum than the other kind. If one finds that drinking sweet wine causes thirst, it does not produce so much sputum as the other kind of wine; if it does not cause thirst, the opposite is true.

51. The main points in favour of and against white strong wine have already been pointed out in the description of sweet wine. As it passes more easily to the bladder than the other kind and is diuretic and purgative, it is always very beneficial in acute diseases. For even though it is less suitable than the sweet in other respects, yet the cleansing through the bladder

which it causes is beneficial so long as it is administered correctly. These are good points to note about the beneficial and the harmful properties of wine; they were unknown to my predecessors.

52. Tawny wine and bitter red wine should be employed in these diseases in this way. If there is neither headache nor affection of the mind, if there is no retention of sputum or urine, and if the stools are rather too loose and full of shreds, it is desirable to change from white or such wines to these. It should also be understood that the more it is diluted, the less harm it will do to the upper organs and to the bladder, while the less it is diluted, the greater is the benefit to the intestines.

53. To drink a mixture of honey and water throughout an illness caused by an acute disease is generally less suitable for those with bitter bile and enlarged viscera than it is for those who have not these things. It is less productive of thirst than is sweet wine and it softens the lung allowing sputum to be brought up in moderation and soothes a cough. It has some detersive quality which makes the sputum less tenacious than it would otherwise be. Hydromel is also a fair diuretic provided that none of the viscera interfere with this action. It also causes the passage of bilious stools, sometimes good ones, but sometimes they are excessive and more frothy than they should be. This is more likely to occur in those who are bilious or have enlargement of the viscera.

54. Softening of the lungs and expectoration of sputum is produced by a greater dilution of honey; frothy stools as well as those which are excessive and warmer than they should be, are due to a less diluted mixture. Stools of this kind bring other considerable troubles. Thus, instead of burning feelings in the hypochondrium being allayed they are provoked and cause distress, tossing of the limbs and ulceration of the internal organs or of the anus. Measures to prevent these things happening will be described.

55. The administration of honey and water without any gruel, instead of any other drink, is more often successful than not in these diseases. Of the reasons why in some cases it

should be given and in some not, the chief points have been stated.

56. Honey and water is generally acknowledged to enfeeble those who drink it and, for this reason, it has acquired a reputation for hastening death. It got this name from people starving to death, as some actually use this mixture for such a purpose. In fact it does not hasten death in all cases but is much more strengthening than water alone so long as it does not upset the stomach. Compared with white wine or with weak or odourless wine, it is some ways more strengthening and in others more weakening. There is a vast difference in the effect on a patient's strength of wine and honey when taken undiluted. If a man were to eat a certain quantity of honey and another were to drink twice as much neat wine, the man who had eaten honey would gain much more strength so long as his stomach were not upset, for the wine causes the passage of much larger stools. If a man were to take gruel and then drink honey and water on top of it, the mixture would be too filling and would cause wind, besides being bad for the organs in the hypochondrium. However, it is not so harmful when drunk before gruel and may even be of some benefit.

57. Boiled hydromel is much more attractive in appearance than is the raw preparation, as it is then sparkling, thin, colourless and transparent. But I cannot attribute to it any other virtue that the raw drink does not possess. It is not even any sweeter than when taken raw, so long as the honey is good. It is, however, weaker and less productive of stools, neither of which are virtues in the case of honey and water. It is best used boiled when the honey is bad, not properly cleared, dark and of ill odour. Cooking will remove the worst of these faults.

58. You will also find the drink known as oxymel useful in these diseases as it promotes the bringing up of sputum and good respiration. The following are some useful points about it. If very sharp, its effect on tenacious sputum will be extreme. If it results in the bringing up of whatever is causing hoarseness and making the throat slippery and, as it were, sweeps the windpipe clean, then it will soothe the lungs owing to its

softening properties. Should all these things happen it is very beneficial. But sometimes for all its sharpness, oxymel fails to win the struggle to bring up the sputum but increases its viscosity and does harm. This is specially liable to happen in those who are in other respects likely to die and are unable to cough and fetch up the matter within. The patient's strength should be estimated with this in mind and, if there is hope, give it. If you do administer oxymel, give it just lukewarm, a little at a time and not in large quantities.

59. On the other hand, oxymel that is only slightly sharp moistens the mouth and pharynx, brings up the sputum and quenches thirst. It is good for the hypochondrium and for the neighbouring viscera. It also neutralizes the harmful effect of honey by correcting its bilious quality. It also breaks up wind and stimulates the passing of urine. However, it causes flabbiness in the lower part of the bowel and the passage of shreds. There are occasions when it is bad for those suffering from acute illnesses especially in that it prevents wind from passing through but makes it come back. It may also enfeeble the patient and chill his limbs. This is the only harm worth mentioning that oxymel can cause, so far as I know.

60. It is advisable to take a little of this drink of oxymel at night and on an empty stomach before taking gruel, though there is nothing to prevent its being taken a good while after the gruel is taken. Those who are subsisting on a completely fluid diet with no gruel will not find it suitable for continued use. This is chiefly because of the scraping and roughening which it produces in the intestines, and if the patient passes no stools it is likely to cause these things while the patient is taking nothing. Then, too, the honey and water might lose some of its strength. Should however the disease as a whole seem to benefit by the copious use of this draught, add only a suspicion of vinegar to the honey. This will avoid the most likely ill-effects and benefit the parts which need it.

61. To sum up, the sharpness obtained from vinegar is more beneficial to those with bitter bile than those with black bile because it dissolves bitter substances, turns them into phlegm and fetches them up. Black bile is lightened, brought up and

diluted, for vinegar brings up black bile. Vinegar is generally more harmful to women than to men as it may cause pains in the womb.

62. There is no virtue which I can attribute to the drinking of water in acute disease. It neither soothes a cough in pneumonia, nor does it promote the expectoration of sputum so well as other drinks, if taken throughout the illness. However, if a little water is taken when changing over from oxymel to hydromel, it brings up the sputum on account of the change in the quality of the drinks by causing a sort of flood. Otherwise it does not even quench thirst but rather causes bitterness because it is of bilious nature, and is thus bad for those of bilious constitution and for the hypochondrium. The worst time to drink it is on an empty stomach for it is then most bilious in its effect and weakening. Water also causes enlargement of the spleen and liver when these are inflamed and it distends the stomach causing indigestion. It passes through slowly because it is both cold and crude and promotes neither the passage of stools nor of urine. This naturally constipating effect may prove harmful. If ever drunk when the feet are cold, it does very great harm to any organ that it attacks.

63. If there is any suspicion of a violent headache or derangement of the mind in these diseases, wine must be completely avoided. In such a case water should be given or, if wine is taken, it should be well watered down and tawny and quite devoid of smell. After such a draught, a small quantity of water should be taken. This prevents the strength of the wine going to the head and affecting the mind. Instructions as to when water alone should be drunk, when in large quantities and when more moderately, when warm and when cold, have already been given in part. The remainder will be mentioned in the appropriate places.

64. Similarly, instructions will be given in dealing with each disease regarding the other drinks that may be taken. The correct indications will be given for giving drinks made from barley, herbs, raisins or the second pressing of grapes, from wheat, thistle or myrtle, pomegranates and the rest. The same applies to compounded drugs.

L

65. Bathing is beneficial to most patients, but the benefit is not always lasting. Sometimes it must be used less than one otherwise would owing to the patient's lack of adequate facilities. There are not many houses where the necessary equipment and servants of the right kind are available. A bath can do no little harm if it is not taken in the right way. A sheltered spot free from smoke is needed, and plenty of water. Baths should be frequent but not excessively so unless there is some special reason. It is better not to be rubbed with soap, but if soap-mixture be used it should be warm and added to the water in far larger quantities than is usually the case and a further generous quantity should be added later and more soon afterwards. The patient should not have far to go to the bath-tub and it should be easy to get in and out of it. The bather should be quiet and orderly and should do nothing for himself; others should pour the water and rub him. A large quantity of tepid water should be prepared and it should quickly be poured over the bather. Sponges are better than scrapers and the body should not be allowed to get too dry before it is anointed. The head however should be dried as well as possible by wiping it with a sponge. Do not allow the extremities, the head and the rest of the body, to become chilled. Do not bathe shortly after food or drink, and do not eat or drink shortly after a bath.

66. The decision whether to bath or not should rest largely with the patient if he is particularly fond of his bath and accustomed to it. Such people are more eager for it and derive benefit from bathing and suffer harm from abstaining. Generally speaking, it is most suitable for the treatment of cases of pneumonia and of *causus*, for bathing soothes pain in the side and chest and in the broad part of the back. It also causes the sputum to ripen and aids its expectoration; it promotes good respiration and relieves fatigue. It also relaxes the joints and softens the skin; it promotes the secretion of urine, cures headache and makes the nose moist.

67. Such then are the beneficial effects of bathing, if all necessities are available. Should however one or more of the necessary accompaniments be lacking, there is a risk that the

bath will do more harm than good, for any one thing can cause considerable harm if it is not previously prepared by the attendants as it should be.

Bathing is least opportune for those suffering from diseases in which the bowels are more relaxed than they should be, nor should patients bathe who are too constipated and have not had any evacuation first.

Baths are also bad for those who are weak, those suffering from nausea or from vomiting, those who are bringing up bilious matter and those who have epistaxis unless this is trivial; you know what is opportune. If the indications are slight, a bath should be taken whether it benefits the whole body or only the head.

68. If then the preparations are satisfactory and the patient welcomes the idea, a bath should be taken every day. It will do no harm to those who are fond of bathing if they take one twice a day. Bathing is much more suitable for those who are on a diet of whole gruel and not just barley-water, though there are times when the latter too may bathe. Least of all should those who take only fluids bathe, though here again it may be allowed in some cases.

A decision must be based on what has been said about the type of patients who will derive benefit or not, according to their regimen. Those who need any of the beneficial effects of bathing should bathe in so far as it benefits them; but in those cases where there is no need of these effects, and any of the signs which renders bathing harmful is present, baths should be avoided.

APHORISMS

The anthology of medical truths which has been famous enough to add a word to the English language.

Section I.

1. Life is short, science is long; opportunity is elusive, experiment is dangerous, judgement is difficult. It is not enough for the physician to do what is necessary, but the patient and the attendants must do their part as well, and circumstances must be favourable.

2. In disturbances of the stomach and when there is spontaneous vomiting, it is beneficial to the patient if the noxious matter be voided. If it is not, then the reverse is the case. Similarly with fasting; if the desired effect be obtained there is benefit, but otherwise it is harmful. Accordingly, the place and season, the age of the patient and the nature of the disease must all be considered.

3. In the case of athletes too good a condition of health is treacherous if it be an extreme state; for it cannot quietly stay as it is, and therefore, since it cannot change for the better, can only change for the worse. For this reason it is well to lose no time in putting an end to such a good condition of health, so that the body can start again to reconstitute itself. Do not allow the body to attain extreme thinness for that too is treacherous, but bring it only to a condition which will naturally continue unchanged, whatever that may be. Likewise fasting, if taken to extremes, is treacherous; and so also is putting on weight, if excessive.

4. A light and frugal dietary is dangerous in chronic complaints and in those acute diseases where it is not indicated. Dieting which causes excessive loss of weight, as well as the feeding up of the emaciated, is beset with difficulties.

5. Sick people are in error when they take a light diet which only increases their distress. Then, whatever be wrong, they only become more ill on a light diet than they would on a

slightly more substantial one. For this reason, light and frugal diets, when persisted in, are dangerous even for the healthy, because the undernourished do not bear an illness so well as the well nourished. Therefore, on the whole, light and frugal diets are more dangerous than those which are a little more substantial.

6. Desperate cases need the most desperate remedies.

7. During the specially acute phase of a disease, pain is most severe and the lightest possible diet is advisable. At other times, when a more substantial diet is permitted, it should be increased slowly in proportion as the seriousness of the disease decreases.

8. When the disease is at its height, then the lightest diet must be employed.

9. It must also be considered whether the patient will be strong enough for the diet prescribed when the disease is at its height. Will the patient be exhausted first and not be strong enough for the diet, or will the disease be blunted and exhausted first?

10. A light diet must be employed from the first in those diseases which rapidly approach their height. But when a disease only gradually attains its maximum severity, the diet need be reduced only then and for a little time before. Previously a richer diet may be employed depending upon the strength of the patient.

11. During a paroxysm the diet must be reduced, for an increase then would be harmful. Thus, in those diseases in which paroxysms occur at intervals, the diet must be reduced at each recrudescence.

12. Paroxysms and periods of remission may be foretold by the nature of the disease. Thus, the season of the year and the periodicity of the paroxysms, whether they be quotidian or tertian or at longer intervals, serve as indications. The signs which appear also assist. For instance, if sputum appear in a case of pleurisy early in the disease, it signifies that the illness will be a short one; if late, that the illness will be prolonged. The appearance of the urine, stools and sweat will also give

some indication of the expected duration and seriousness of a malady.

13. Old people bear fasting most easily, then adults, much less youths and least of all children. The more active they are, the less do they bear it.

14. Things which are growing have the greatest natural warmth and, accordingly, need most nourishment. Failing this, the body becomes exhausted. Old men have little warmth and they need little food which produces warmth; too much only extinguishes the warmth they have. For this reason, fevers are not so acute in old people for then the body is cold.

15. In winter and spring, stomachs are warm and sleep longest. Accordingly, more food should be given in these seasons, for the body produces more warmth and thus needs more nourishment. Young men and athletes show the truth of this.

16. Fluid diets are beneficial to all who suffer from fevers, but this is specially true in the case of children and the edentulous who are accustomed to such kind of food.

17. In deciding whether food should be given once or twice a day, more often or less, in greater or in smaller quantities at a time, one must consider habit, age, place and season.

18. Farinaceous food is most difficult to digest in summer and autumn, easiest in winter and next easiest in spring.

19. In those maladies where paroxysms occur at intervals, give no food just before the paroxysm nor compel the patient to take anything, but reduce his usual diet.

20. When a disease has attained the crisis, or when a crisis has just passed, do not disturb the patient with innovation in treatment either by the administration of drugs or by giving stimulants. Let them be.

21. The progress of a disease should be so guided, where guidance is needed, so that it develops in the most favourable manner according to its natural tendency.

22. Use drugs only when the disease for which you employ them has come to a head and not when it is developing, unless it be ripe for such treatment, which is rarely the case.

23. Do not judge the stools by their quantity but by their

quality and the manner of them, what is needful and comfortable for the patient. Where it is necessary to bring the patient
to a fainting condition, even this should be done, if he be
strong enough to stand it.

24. In acute diseases employ drugs very seldom and only at
the beginning. Even then, never prescribe them until you
have made a thorough examination of the patient.

25. If what ought to be voided is voided, it is beneficial and
easily borne by the patient; if not, it is borne with difficulty.

Section II.

1. A disease in which sleep causes trouble is fatal. Where
sleep is beneficial, it is not fatal.

2. Sleep that stops delirium is good.

3. Both sleep and wakefulness are bad if they exceed their
due proportion.

4. Neither a surfeit of food nor of fasting is good, nor
anything else which exceeds the measure of nature.

5. Unprovoked fatigue means disease.

6. Those who are suffering from a bodily malady and do not
feel much of the pain of it, are also suffering from mental
disease.

7. When bodies become thin over a long period of time,
feed them up again slowly. But when the wasting has come
on in a short time, feed them up again quickly.

8. If, subsequent to an illness, a patient does not derive
strength from the nourishment he takes, it means he requires
more food. But if this happens when adequate nourishment is
taken, it means a purge is necessary.

9. When it is desired to purge, the aim should be an easy
evacuation.

10. The more nourishment you give to a person who has
not been purged, the more harm you do.

11. It is better to be full of drink than full of food.

12. What is left behind in the body after the crisis frequently
causes relapse.

13. A patient finds the night before a crisis trying, but the
succeeding night is generally more comfortable.

14. In the case of haemorrhage from the stomach, a change in the character of the stool, if not clearly unfavourable, may indicate a change for the better.

15. Examine the stool in the case of patients suffering from diseases of the throat or from tumours of the body. If it be bilious, the disease is part of a sickness of the whole body. But if it resembles a normal stool, then the disease is localized and it is safe to feed the body.

16. Hard work is undesirable for the underfed.

17. Over-eating causes sickness, as the cure shows.

18. Those who eat their food quickly in large pieces, quickly void it.

19. It is unwise to prophesy either death or recovery in acute diseases.

20. Those who have relaxed bowels when they are young have constipated ones in later life; but if their bowels are constipated in youth they become relaxed as they grow old.

21. Hunger is alleviated by the drinking of neat wine.

22. Disease which results from over-eating is cured by fasting; disease following fasting, by a surfeit. So with other things; cures may be effected by opposites.

23. Acute diseases attain the crisis within fourteen days.

24. In the progress of a disease, it is the fourth day in each period of seven days which is indicative. Taking the eighth day of the disease as the beginning of the second period of seven days, it is the eleventh day which must be observed since that is the fourth day of the second period. Again, the eighteenth day must be watched since this is the fourth day after the fourteenth or the seventh after the eleventh.

25. In summer, quartan fevers are usually of short duration; in autumn they last long, especially those contracted when winter is near.

26. It is better that a fever should succeed a convulsion than a convulsion follow a fever.

27. Too much hope must not be put in the regression of a disease when this happens without obvious cause, neither should deterioration occurring contrary to expectation be

feared overmuch. Such changes are of uncertain significance and usually last but a short time.

28. In feverish illnesses it is bad either if the body remains superficially the same and does not waste, or if it wastes more than might be expected. In the former case the malady will be long; in the latter there is evidence of the patient weakening.

29. Purge at the start of an illness if you think fit, but, when a disease is at its height, it is better to withhold such action.

30. Everything is at its weakest at the beginning and at the end, but strongest at its height.

31. It is a bad thing if a patient does not put on weight when he is being fed up after an illness.

32. As a general rule, if those who are poorly take their food well at first, but fail to put on weight, they finish by refusing food. On the other hand, if they firmly refuse food at first but take it later on, they make a good recovery.

33. In every illness, a healthy frame of mind and an eager application to victuals is good. The reverse is bad.

34. There is less danger from a disease which is proper to the nature, condition and age of a patient, or to the time of year, than if it be not proper to one of these.

35. In all maladies, those who are fat about the belly do best; it is bad to be very thin and wasted there. Purging may be dangerous in the latter case.

36. Those who are in unhealthy bodily condition are very liable to faint from the administration of purgative drugs, as do those who do not take the right food.

37. Those who are in good bodily condition are hard to purge.

38. With regard to food and drink, it is better to take something slightly less suitable but pleasing than something more suitable but less pleasing.

39. The old feel ill less often than the young, but when they contract chronic ailments these usually accompany them to the grave.

40. Hoarseness and running of the nose do not 'ripen' in the very old.

41. Those who are subject to frequent and severe fainting attacks without obvious cause die suddenly.

42. It is impossible to cure a severe attack of apoplexy and no easy matter to cure a mild one.

43. Those who have been strangled and who are unconscious but not yet dead will not recover if there is foam about the lips.

44. Sudden death is more common in those who are naturally fat than in the lean.

45. The chief factor in the cure of epilepsy in the young is change, especially that due to growing up, but seasonal change of climate, or change of place or mode of life are also important.

46. If a patient be subject to two pains arising in different parts of the body simultaneously, the stronger blunts the other.

47. Pain and fever are more marked while pus is forming than when it is formed.

48. Rest, as soon as there is pain, is a great restorative in all disturbances of the body.

49. Those who are used to bearing an accustomed pain, even if they be weak and old, bear it more easily than the young and strong who are unaccustomed.

50. What has become customary by long endurance is wont to give less annoyance than what is not customary, even if the former be more severe. But it may sometimes be necessary to produce a change to what is unaccustomed.

51. It is dangerous to disturb the body violently whether it be by starvation or by feeding, by making it hot or cold, or in any way whatsoever. All excesses are inimical to nature. It is safer to proceed a little at a time, especially when changing from one regimen to another.

52. If you apply all the regular treatment without getting the regular result, do not therefore change the treatment so long as your original diagnosis remains unchanged.

53. Those who have relaxed bowels, if they are young, tend to do better than those with constipated ones, but worse if they are getting old; for it is a general rule that the bowels become constipated with advancing years.

54. A heavy physique is noble and not unpleasing in the young; in old age it is awkward and less desirable than a smaller stature.

Section III.

1. The changes of the seasons are especially liable to beget diseases, as are great changes from heat to cold, or cold to heat in any season. Other changes in the weather have similarly severe effects.

2. Some natures are naturally well-suited to summer and some to winter; others are ill-suited to one or the other.

3. Diseases vary in their relationships one with another; some are opposed, some are mutually agreeable. Similarly, certain ages are well or ill-suited to certain seasons, places and regimens.

4. When cold and heat both occur on the same day at any time of the year, then you must expect those diseases commonly encountered in autumn.

5. South winds cause deafness, misty vision, headache, sluggishness and a relaxed condition of the body. When this wind is prevalent these symptoms occur in illnesses. The north wind brings coughs, sore throats, constipation, retention of urine accompanied by rigors, pains in the sides and breast. When this wind is prevalent such things will be encountered among the sick.

6. When the summer is spring-like in character, then expect great diaphoresis in the course of fevers.

7. During periods of drought fevers are high. If the whole year be mainly dry, whatever the general climatic condition produced, expect similar illnesses.

8. When the weather is seasonable and the crops ripen at the regular times, diseases are regular in their appearance and easily reach their crisis. When the weather is irregular, diseases are irregular and their crises difficult.

9. It is in autumn that diseases tend to be most acute and most likely to prove fatal. The spring is the healthiest and least fatal time of year.

10. Autumn is best for consumptives.

11. As regards the seasons: a dry winter with northerly winds followed by a wet spring and southerly winds produces acute fevers, ophthalmia and dysentery in the summer. This is specially true of women and those of a watery constitution.

12. On the other hand, a damp mild winter accompanied by southerly winds, followed by a dry spring in which the wind is from the north, tends to produce miscarriage on the slightest pretext in women approaching term in the spring. If parturition is accomplished the children are weak and sickly, so that either the children die at once or, should they survive, they are thin and fall ill frequently. This same character of the seasons gives rise to dysentery and dry ophthalmia as well, while the aged suffer from catarrh which may speedily prove fatal.

13. A dry summer accompanied by northerly winds and a wet autumn with southerly winds produce during the following winter headaches, coughs, hoarseness, running at the nose and, in some cases, wasting.

14. Alternatively, a rainless autumn in which the winds come from the north is advantageous to women and those of a watery diathesis. Others suffer from dry ophthalmia, from acute fevers, from running at the nose and, in some cases, from melancholy.

15. As regards the weather in general: drought is more healthy than rain and less likely to provoke fatal illness.

16. The diseases usually peculiar to rainy periods are chronic fevers, diarrhoea, gangrene, epilepsy, apoplexy and sore throats. Those peculiar to a time of drought are consumption, ophthalmia, arthritis, strangury and dysentery.

17. As for the daily changes in the weather: a north wind stimulates the body and makes it of good tone and agile, and makes for a good complexion and acuity of hearing; the bowels are constipated and the eyes sting. But a pain in the chest is made worse by such a wind. On the other hand, south winds relax the body, make the tissues moist, reduce acuity of hearing and produce headaches and vertigo. Movement both of the eyes and of the body generally is sluggish and the bowels relaxed.

18. As for the seasons, in spring and full summer children

and young people do best; in summer and, up to a point, autumn, the old; while the winter suits best those between these two groups.

19. Every disease occurs at all seasons of the year but some of them more frequently occur and are of greater severity at certain times.

20. For example, madness, melancholy, epilepsy, haemorrhages, sore throats, catarrh, hoarseness, coughs, leprosy, vitiligo, ulcerative eruptions—these are very common—tumours and arthritis are all common in the spring.

21. In summer, while some of the foregoing occur, we must also expect continued fevers, *causus*, tertian fevers, vomiting, diarrhoea, ophthalmia, earache, buccal ulcers, gangrene of the genitalia and heat spots.

22. In autumn, while we still encounter many of the summer ailments, you must expect as well quartan fevers, irregular fevers, diseases of the spleen, dropsy, consumption, strangury, enteritis, dysentery, pains in the hips, sore throats, ileus, epilepsy, madness and melancholy.

23. During the winter season, pleurisy, pneumonia, lethargy, catarrh of the nose, hoarseness, cough, pain in the chest, pains in the side and loins, headaches, vertigo and apoplexy all occur.

24. Then, if diseases be grouped according to different ages we find that new-born infants suffer from aphthae, vomiting, cough, insomnia, nightmares, inflammation of the umbilicus and discharging ears.

25. When teething takes place, we must add painful gums, fevers, convulsions and diarrhoea. These are specially to be expected during the eruption of the canines and in plump children or those with hard bellies.

26. As they grow older, tonsilitis, retro-pharyngeal abscesses, asthma, stone, infection with round worms and ascaris, pedunculated warts, priapism, scrofulous swellings in the cervical glands and other tumours are seen.

27. On approaching puberty, besides the foregoing diseases we must add long-continued fevers and epistaxis.

28. Usually children's diseases reach the crisis either in forty days, in seven lunar months or in seven years. Others resolve

on the approach of puberty. However, should a disease persist after puberty or, in the case of girls, the time when menstruation is established, it is likely to become chronic.

29. In youths, haemoptysis, consumption, acute fevers and epilepsy besides other ailments must be added, but especially those mentioned above.

30. Later, we encounter asthma, pleurisy, pneumonia, lethargy, inflammation of the brain, *causus*, chronic diarrhoea, cholera, dysentery, enteritis and haemorrhoids.

31. In the old, dyspnoea, catarrhal coughs, strangury, dysuria, arthritis, nephritis, dizziness, apoplexy, cachexia, pruritus of the whole body, insomnia, ascites and fluid in the eyes and nostrils, failing sight, blindness from glaucoma and deafness.

Section IV.

1. Drugs may be administered to pregnant women from the fourth to the seventh month of gestation. After that period, the dose should be less. Care must also be exercised in giving drugs to infants and children.

2. Drugs should be used to evacuate from the body such substances which, should they flow of their own accord, would be beneficial. Those substances, evacuation of which would not be advantageous, should be stopped from coming.

3. If those substances are purged which ought to be purged, it is beneficial and the patient bears it well; if the reverse, it is borne ill.

4. In summer-time, use drugs acting rather on the upper part of the bowel; in winter the lower part.

5. The administration of drugs is attended with difficulty at the rising of the Dog Star and shortly before.

6. Thin subjects who are prone to vomiting should be given medicine for the upper bowel, but reduce the dose in winter.

7. The well-covered, who are not prone to vomiting, should be given drugs for the lower bowel, but in this case avoid the summer.

8. In purging consumptive patients, employ only small doses.

9. The bowel should be treated in melancholics by the same reasoning applying the opposite treatment.

10. In very acute conditions, administer the required drugs on the same day as they are shown to be required. It is bad for such conditions to last long.

11. Patients suffering from colicky pains about the navel and aching in the loins develop distension unless the malady is dispersed by drugs or by other means.

12. It is bad to administer drugs acting on the small bowel during the winter in patients prone to enteritis.

13. Patients in whom purgation of the upper bowel is attended with difficulty should have their bodies moistened beforehand by administering more food and giving more rest, before the prescription of hellebore.

14. When anyone takes a draught of hellebore, he should be made to move about rather than left to rest and sleep. Sea travel demonstrates the efficacy of movement in producing a disturbance of the intestines.

15. If you wish hellebore to act more efficiently, keep the patient moving. When you wish to stop its action, order rest and sleep.

16. Hellebore is a dangerous drug for those with healthy flesh since in these it induces convulsions.

17. A patient without fever and no appetite who suffers from heartburn, vertigo and bitterness in the mouth requires medicine for the upper part of the body.

18. Pain above the diaphragm indicates the need for drugs acting on the upper part of the body; pain below, for those acting on the belly.

19. When a purge is given to a patient who is not thirsty, its action continues until he becomes thirsty.

20. If an afebrile patient suffers from colic, heaviness of the legs and aching in the loins, he needs drugs for the lower organs.

21. Black excrement, like blood, appearing spontaneously has a serious significance whether it be accompanied by fever or not. The darker it is the more serious the condition. But

when dark stools are due to drugs, however dark the colour, it is of little significance.

22. The vomiting or passage of dark bile at the beginning of an illness is fatal.

23. Those who show great wasting, either from acute or chronic illness or from wounds, and then pass dark bile or something resembling black blood, die the next day.

24. Dysentery starting with the passage of black blood is fatal.

25. The vomiting of blood of any kind is bad; its passage as excrement is not a good sign, as is the passage of black stools.

26. Cases of dysentery in which pieces resembling solid tissue appear in the stools are fatal.

27. If a fever be attended with considerable haemorrhage from any part of the body, the patient's bowels become relaxed during recovery.

28. Biliousness of the stool ceases upon the supervention of deafness, deafness upon the appearance of bilious excrement.

29. A rigor occurring on the sixth day of a fever is a sign of a dangerous crisis.

30. A paroxysm which appears at the same hour on one day as it departed on the previous day is a sign of a crisis.

31. Suppurative inflammations about the joints, especially about the jaws, may follow exhaustion from fevers.

32. During recovery from an illness, pain about a part indicates that suppuration will occur there.

33. But should pain in a part have existed before the onset of the disease, then that is the site where the malady establishes itself.

34. Sudden choking without swelling of the throat in a patient with fever leads to a fatal outcome.

35. If the neck be suddenly twisted round and swallowing becomes almost impossible in a patient showing no swelling, then he will die.

36. Paroxysms of sweating in the course of fevers occurring on the 3rd, 5th, 7th, 9th, 11th, 14th, 17th, 21st, 27th, 31st and 34th days of the disease are of good omen. Such paroxysms

mark the crisis of the disease. But should such paroxysms not occur, then expect pain, a long illness and relapse.

37. In severe fevers, cold paroxysms of sweating indicate death; in milder cases a long illness.

38. The appearance of sweat on a particular part of the body indicates disease in that part.

39. Should one part of the body be hotter or colder than the rest, disease is present in that part.

40. Variation in the condition of the body, if it becomes cold and then hot again, or changes colour, indicates a long illness.

41. Severe sweating after sleep without obvious cause signifies that the body has too much nourishment. If it happens that the patient is not taking his food, then he needs purging.

42. Continued sweating, whether hot or cold, indicates disease. If the body be cold, it is a major illness; if hot, a minor.

43. Fevers which do not intermit but which increase each alternate day are dangerous. Intermission, of whatever kind, shows that the malady is not dangerous.

44. Prolonged fevers may give rise to swelling and pains in the joints.

45. Those suffering from swelling and pain in the joints are taking too much food.

46. When a rigor supervenes on an unremitting fever when the patient has already been weakened, the outcome is fatal.

47. Livid, bloody, foul-smelling or bilious sputum supervening in cases of continued fever is of bad significance. However, if such expectoration remove the diseased tissues, all may be well. A similar rule applies to the urine and to the stools. But unless separation occurs properly through these parts the outlook is poor.

48. Cold skin associated with a high internal temperature and thirst in a patient with continued fever is fatal.

49. In a continued fever, if the lip, eyebrow, eye or nostril be distorted; if the patient, being already weak, does not see

M

or does not hear—if any of these things happen, death is at hand.

50. If, in a continued fever, respiration becomes difficult and delirium occurs, expect a fatal outcome.

51. Unless an abscess associated with fever discharge about the time of the first crises, a long illness is to be expected.

52. There is nothing strange in those suffering from fevers, or from other illness, deliberately weeping. But if they weep spontaneously, in spite of themselves, it is of more significance.

53. When, in fevers, the gums suppurate, the fever is increased.

54. In fevers of the type of *causus* where there is a frequent dry cough irritating slightly, thirst is not produced.

55. Fevers lasting more than one day which follow on a bubo are all serious.

56. A paroxysm of sweating in the course of a fever which is not associated with a fall in temperature is of bad significance. It indicates excess of moisture in the body and the illness will be prolonged.

57. Fever succeeding a convulsion or tetanus, ends the illness.

58. An attack of shivering supervening in a case of *causus* puts an end to it.

59. A pure tertian fever reaches its crisis after a maximum of seven paroxysms.

60. When in the course of a fever, deafness, epistaxis or disorder of the stomach supervenes, the illness is approaching its end.

61. If the length of a fever is not an odd number of days, relapse is likely to occur.

62. If jaundice appears in a case of fever in less than seven days, the outlook is bad unless watery discharges from the belly occur.

63. In fevers attended with daily rigors, the fever intermits daily; it is not remittent.

64. Jaundice occurring on the 7th, 9th, 11th or 14th day of a fever is favourable unless the right hypochondrium be hard. In other cases, the outlook is unfavourable.

65. A sensation of burning in the belly and heartburn are of bad significance in fevers.

66. In acute fevers convulsions or violent pains in the intestines are of bad significance.

67. In cases of fever, fears on waking from sleep, or convulsions, are serious.

68. Irregular breathing in cases of fever is bad since it indicates a fit.

69. When the urine of a man with fever is thick, full of clots and of small quantity, an increase in quantity and clarity is advantageous. Such a change is especially likely to occur if, from the beginning or very shortly afterwards, the urine has a sediment.

70. Those whose urine during a fever is turbid like that of a beast of burden either suffer from headache or will do so.

71. When the crisis of an illness is reached on the seventh day, the urine shows a red cloud on the fourth day and is otherwise normal.

72. Colourless urine is bad; it is specially common in those with disease of the brain.

73. If pain in the loins and fever supervene when the hypochondrium is distended and full of rumblings, the bowels become relaxed unless wind breaks or the patient passes a large quantity of urine.

74. When suppuration is suspected in a joint, the suppuration is avoided if the urine which flows is thick and white, like that which is seen sometimes in wearisome quartan fevers.

75. Blood or pus in the urine indicates ulceration of the kidneys or of the bladder.

76. Small fleshy objects, the shape of hairs, in the urine which is thick, mean there is a discharge from the kidneys.

77. Thick urine containing bran-like particles indicates inflammation of the bladder.

78. The sudden appearance of blood in the urine indicates that a small renal vessel has burst.

79. A sandy urinary sediment shows that a stone is forming in the bladder.

80. When blood clots in the urine are accompanied by

strangury, abdominal and perineal pain, it is the perivesicular tissues which are affected.

81. The presence of blood, pus and flakes in a foul-smelling urine indicates an ulcer of the bladder.

82. If a tumour form in the urethra, suppuration and discharge of the abscess produces resolution.

83. Much urine passed at night means a small stool.

Section V.

1. Convulsions following the administration of hellebore are fatal.

2. Convulsions succeeding upon a wound are fatal.

3. When a convulsion or a fit of hiccoughs follows severe haemorrhage, the outlook is bad.

4. A convulsion or a fit of hiccoughs following excessive purging is bad.

5. If a drunk man suddenly becomes speechless in a fit, he will die after convulsions unless a fever ensue or unless, upon recovering from his hangover, he regains his voice.

6. Unless those who contract tetanus die within four days they recover.

7. Those who suffer from epilepsy in childhood recover from it, but when it first appears after the age of twenty-five it usually continues till death.

8. If sufferers from pleurisy do not cough up material within fourteen days, the inflammation produces empyema.

9. Consumption occurs most frequently between the ages of eighteen and thirty-five.

10. Those in whom, from a sore throat, the disease passes to the lungs, either die within seven days or, surviving this period, suffer from empyema.

11. If the sputum of those suffering from consumption have an unpleasant smell when poured on hot coals and if the hairs fall from the head, a fatal outcome results.

12. In consumption, loss of the hair of the head accompanied by diarrhoea is fatal.

13. Frothy blood comes from the lungs.

14. Diarrhoea supervening on consumption is a fatal sign.

15. If those patients in which pleurisy has resulted in empyema evacuate the abscess by expectoration within forty days following its bursting, they recover. If this is not so, they become consumptive.

16. Frequent over-heating of the body causes the following troubles: relaxation of the flesh, nervous weakness, benumbing of the mind, haemorrhage, fainting attacks and in some cases death.

17. Cold causes fits, tetanus, gangrene and febrile shivering fits.

18. Cold is bad for the bones, teeth, nerves and the spinal cord; heat is good for these structures.

19. Parts that have been chilled should be thoroughly warmed unless there is bleeding or the likelihood of this.

20. In patients already suffering from ulcers, cold is of severe effect. It hardens the flesh round about, causes pain without suppuration, gangrene, feverish rigors, spasms and tetanus.

21. In young, well nourished people, tetanus is sometimes seen which does not follow upon an ulcer. In these a cold douche in summer produces a reaction of warmth and this warmth effects a cure.

22. Warmth which produces suppuration, as it may do with some but not all ulcers, is an important sign of recovery. It softens the tissues, dries them up and relieves pain. Further, rigors, spasms and tetanus are resolved. To the head, it relieves headaches. Warmth is also of value in the treatment of broken bones, especially when the bone is exposed. It is useful in the treatment of ulcers on the head. Those parts of the body where ulcers or gangrene have been caused by exposure to cold benefit much from warmth and a crisis is attained. Similar advantage from warmth is observed in cases of ulceration of the anus, the private parts, the womb and the bladder. Cold, in these diseases, is inimical and killing.

23. Cold should be applied in the following cases: when there is haemorrhage or the danger of one. In such cases apply the cold not to the actual spot from which bleeding occurs or is expected, but round about. Cold should also be applied to

boils or pustules when these tend to be red or suffused with fresh blood. Cold turns pustules dark when they are long-standing. Cold applications are also indicated in cases of erysipelas where there is no ulceration; if ulcers have formed it is harmful.

24. Cold substances such as snow and ice are harmful to the chest; they cause cough, haemorrhage and fluxes.

25. Swelling and pain in the joints unassociated with ulceration, gout and spasms, are mostly relieved and reduced by cold douches and the pain thus dispelled. A moderate numbness relieves pain.

26. Water that is capable of quick heating and quick cooling is very light.

27. When a patient feels thirsty at night and has a great desire to drink and if afterwards he sleep, it is a good sign.

28. Aromatic vapour baths are useful in the treatment of female disorders and would often be useful for other conditions too if they did not cause headaches.

30.[1] Acute diseases are fatal to pregnant women.

31. Miscarriage follows blood-letting in pregnant women, especially if the foetus be large.

32. If a woman vomits blood, this ceases with the onset of menstruation.

33. It is a good sign if epistaxis occurs in a woman whose menstruation has stopped.

34. Frequent diarrhoea in a pregnant woman renders her liable to a miscarriage.

35. When a woman who is afflicted with hysteria, or who is in difficult labour, sneezes, it should be regarded as a good sign.

36. When a woman suffers from leucorrhoea and the discharges do not occur regularly, it is a sign that a purge is required.

37. If the breasts of a pregnant woman regress suddenly, it means she will have a miscarriage.

38. If, in a woman who is carrying twins, one breast becomes thin, a miscarriage will occur of one of the children.

[1] 29 (= IV, 1) is here omitted.

If the right breast is affected, the male child will be lost; if the left, the female.

39. If a woman who is neither pregnant nor has given birth produce milk, her menstruation has stopped.

40. It is a sign of madness when blood congeals about a woman's nipples.

41. To know whether a woman be pregnant, administer a draught of hydromel on retiring when she has had no supper. If she suffers from colic in the stomach she is pregnant; if not, she is not pregnant.

42. A pregnant woman is of good complexion if the child be male; of ill complexion if the child be female.

43. If a pregnant woman have erysipelas of the womb she will die.

44. Pregnant women who are abnormally delicate have a miscarriage before the fœtus becomes sizeable.

45. When women of medium build have miscarriages at two or three months without obvious cause, it is because the placenta is full of mucus. It is thus unable to hold the weight of the fœtus which therefore is ejected.

46. When abnormally fat women do not conceive, it is because the omentum is pressing on the mouth of the uterus. Until they become thin, they do not become pregnant.

47. If suppuration in the womb spreads to the region round the hip joint, lint pledgets should be used to stop it.

48. A male fœtus inclines to the right, a female to the left.

49. When a drug which causes sneezing is used to expel the after-birth, stop up the mouth and nostrils.

50. To restrain a woman's menstruation, apply the largest possible cupping-glass to the nipples.

51. During pregnancy the mouth of the womb is closed.

52. If much milk flow from the breasts of a pregnant woman it means that the fœtus is weak; but if the breasts be dry, the fœtus is healthy.

53. When abortion is threatened the breasts become lax. If the nipples should become hard again, there will be pain in the nipples or in the hip joints or in the eyes or in the knees and abortion will not take place.

54. If the mouth of the womb is hard, it inevitably closes.

55. Pregnant women who catch fevers, or who become very emaciated without obvious cause, either have difficult and dangerous labours or run the risk of miscarriage.

56. A spasm or an attack of fainting following on menstruation is bad.

57. Both menorrhagia and amenorrhoea indicate disease of the womb.

58. Inflammation of the rectum and of the womb produce strangury, as also do suppurative conditions of the kidneys. Inflammation of the liver, however, causes hiccough.

59. If a woman has not conceived and you wish to determine whether conception be possible, wrap her up in a cloak underneath which incense should be burned. If the odour seems to pass through the body to the nose and mouth, then she is not sterile.

60. Menstrual bleeding which occurs during pregnancy indicates an unhealthy fœtus.

61. When a woman who is suffering from neither rigors nor fever develops amenorrhoea and is liable to nausea, she is pregnant.

62. Women in whom the cervical os is cold and thick tend not to conceive easily. Similarly, a very moist os drowns and destroys the semen while an unusually dry and hot condition destroys the seed from lack of nourishment. Women who are free from these extremes are those who conceive best.

63. It is much the same with males. Either the general laxness of the body is such that the inner pressure of the wind is insufficient to eject the semen, or, on account of the thickness of the tissues, adequate moisture does not pass through. Also, excess of coldness or excess of heat will prevent conception.

64. Milk is not recommended for those who suffer from headaches. It is bad, too, for patients with fever, those whose bellies are distended and full of rumbling and those who are thirsty. It is bad also for patients with acute fevers in whom the stools are bilious, and for those who have lost much blood in the stool. It is good for patients liable to consumption if they have not too high a fever. It should also be given in

cases with prolonged low fever, where the patient is abnormally wasted, provided none of the above-mentioned contra-indications is present.

65. Those who suffer from wounds with swelling in addition are not particularly liable to spasms or madness. However, if the swellings suddenly disappear, spasms and tetanus occur where the lesions are situated posteriorly. If, however, the lesions are on the front of the body, acute pain in the sides or suppuration follows. Where the swellings are particularly red, dysentery is seen.

66. If swelling does not occur as a result of serious deep wounds, the outlook is very bad.

67. Loose soft elastic swellings are not serious; hard indurated swellings are serious.

68. When there is pain at the back of the head, some help may be given by dividing the vessel which runs vertically in the forehead.

69. Rigors in women usually begin in the loins and pass through the back to the head. In men they tend to begin in the back, rather than in the front of the body, for instance in the thighs or forearms. But men have a porous skin, as is shown by the hairs.

70. Those who catch quartan fevers are not at all liable to spasms. Should they previously have a spasm and then develop a quartan fever, then the spasms stop.

71. Those whose skin is dry and taut die without sweating. Those whose skin is relaxed and porous die sweating.

72. Jaundiced patients suffer especially from flatulence.

Section VI.

1. In cases of chronic enteritis, the occurrence of heartburn, should it not have occurred before, is a good sign.

2. Those whose noses tend to run and whose semen is watery tend to be rather sickly. Those in whom the reverse is true are healthier.

3. Loss of appetite is bad for long-standing cases of dysentery and particularly when the disease is accompanied by fever.

4. Ulcers with a peeling edge are malignant.

5. Care must be taken to determine whether there are any striking points about the site of any pains complained of; whether they are in the side, in the breast or anywhere else.

6. Diseases of the kidneys and of the bladder are difficult to cure in the aged.

7. Of those pains and swellings which occur in the belly, those which are on the surface are less serious than those which are not.

8. Ulcers on the body are difficult to heal in dropsical patients.

9. Widespread exanthems are not accompanied by much itching.

10. Severe headaches are cured should there be a flow of pus, blood or fluid from the nostrils, mouth or ears.

11. It is good when haemorrhoids supervene on cases of melancholy or where there is renal disease.

12. Where long-standing haemorrhoids have been cured there is danger of dropsy or of wasting supervening unless one be left untreated.

13. Sneezing supervening on an attack of hiccoughs relieves that condition.

14. When, in a case of dropsy, water flows from the blood vessels into the abdominal cavity, the oedema is relieved.

15. Unprovoked vomiting puts an end to long-continued cases of diarrhoea.

16. Diarrhoea supervening in cases of pleurisy or pneumonia is a bad sign.

17. It is good when sufferers from ophthalmia have diarrhoea.

18. Deep wounds of the bladder, brain, heart, diaphragm, of any of the delicate entrails, the stomach or liver are fatal.

19. Division of bone, cartilage, nerve, the delicate part of the jaw, or of the foreskin is not followed by growing and joining together again.

20. Haemorrhage into the abdominal cavity is necessarily followed by suppuration.

21. Varicose veins or haemorrhoids appearing in a case of madness put an end to it.

22. Abscesses extending from the shoulders to the elbows are cured by bleeding.

23. Patients with fear or depression of long standing are subject to melancholia.

24. Division of the delicate entrails is not followed by repair.

25. When erysipelas, beginning on the surface, extends deeply into the body it is bad. However, deep inflammation coming to the surface is good.

26. Trembling in cases of *causus* is cured by delirium.

27. Should surgery or cauterization in patients with ulcers or with dropsy result in the loss of a great quantity of pus or watery fluid, death invariably follows.

28. Eunuchs are not subject to gout, nor do they become bald.

29. Gout does not occur in women except after the menopause.

30. A youth does not suffer from gout until after sexual intercourse.

31. Pains in the eyes are cured by drinking neat wine, by bathing, by vapour baths, by bleeding or by the administration of certain drugs.

32. People who lisp are especially liable to prolonged diarrhoea.

33. Those who suffer from heartburn are not particularly liable to pleurisy.

34. Those who are bald do not suffer from varicose veins, while should someone who is bald develop such veins, then his hair grows again.

35. It is bad when people with dropsy develop a cough, but good if they have the cough before the dropsy starts.

36. Dysuria is cured by bleeding and the incision should be in the inner vein.

37. In a case of sore throat, the development of swellings on the outer aspect of the trachea is a good sign.

38. It is better not to treat those who have internal cancers since, if treated, they die quickly; but if not treated they last a long time.

39. Spasms are cured either by over-eating or by fasting. The same is true of hiccoughs.

40. Pain around the hypochondrium, unattended by inflammation, is relieved by the onset of fever.

41. The thickness of the tissues themselves may be responsible for the absence of the signs of suppuration when the abscess is a deep one.

42. In cases of jaundice it is a bad sign when the liver becomes hard.

43. Should a splenetic patient catch dysentery and this become chronic, dropsy or enteritis supervenes and they die.

44. Those who suffer from anuria as a result of strangury die within seven days unless, a fever supervening, a sufficient flow of urine is re-established.

45. Ulcers lasting a year or longer cause the underlying bone to be eaten away and the resulting scars are depressed.

46. Those who develop a kyphosis from asthma or from cough before reaching puberty, die.

47. In cases where such treatment is advantageous, bleeding or purging is more efficacious in the spring.

48. To catch dysentery is helpful to splenetic patients.

49. The inflammation in all cases of gout subsides within forty days.

50. Laceration of the brain is invariably followed by fever and bilious vomiting.

51. Those in health who are suddenly taken with headache, loss of voice and who show stertorous breathing die within a week unless a fever supervene.

52. Observe the appearance of the eyes during sleep. Should any of the white be visible when the eyelids are closed, provided this be not due to diarrhoea or the taking of a drug, it is a sorry symptom and exceedingly fatal.

53. Raving delirium which is accompanied by laughter is safer; that accompanied by seriousness is more dangerous.

54. Respiration characterized by a sobbing sound in acute febrile illnesses is a bad sign.

55. Gout is usually most active in spring and autumn.

56. In melancholic diseases, a flow of humours to one part

of the body is dangerous in that either apoplexy, a fit, madness or blindness will follow.

57. Apoplexy usually occurs between the ages of forty and sixty.

58. If the mesentery protrude, it invariably rots away.

59. If, in some condition, the hip-joint is dislocated and subsequently reduced again, fluid is formed.

60. If, following chronic pains in the hip, the joint becomes dislocated, the leg wastes away and the patient becomes lame. This may be prevented by the use of the cautery.

Section VII.

1. It is a bad sign in acute illnesses when the extremities become cold.

2. It is a bad sign when the flesh becomes livid in the neighbourhood of a diseased bone.

3. It is bad when vomiting is followed by hiccough and blood-shot eyes.

4. Shuddering succeeding on sweating is not good.

5. It is a good thing in cases of madness when dysentery, dropsy or an ecstatic state supervenes.

6. In prolonged illnesses, anorexia and unadulterated excreta are bad.

7. A shivering fit and delirium following excessive drinking is bad.

8. The bursting of a tumour internally is accompanied by faintness, vomiting and swooning.

9. It is bad when delirium or spasms follow haemorrhage.

10. It is bad when vomiting, hiccough, fits or delirium be observed in a case of ileus.

11. It is bad when pneumonia supervenes upon pleurisy.

12. It is bad when inflammation of the brain supervenes upon pneumonia.

13. Fits or tetanus complicating severe burns are bad.

14. Shock or delirium following a blow on the head is bad.

15. It is bad when purulent sputum follows haemoptysis.

16. The production of purulent sputum is followed by consumption. When the sputum ceases, the patient dies.

17. Hiccough is a bad sign in cases of hepatitis.

18. A convulsion or delirium following insomnia is bad.

18a. Trembling following lethargy is bad.

19. Inflammation of the tissues following exposure of bone is bad.

20. Erysipelas followed by gangrene or by suppuration is bad.

21. When haemorrhage follows ulcers which throb violently, it is bad.

22. Long-standing pain in the belly followed by suppuration is bad.

23. Unmixed stools followed by dysentery are bad.

24. Delirium follows the fracture of a bone if the ends are not in apposition.

25. A convulsion following the administration of a drug is fatal.

26. It is bad when, following violent abdominal pains, the extremities become cold.

27. In the case of pregnant women, straining at stool may bring about miscarriage.

28. Bones, cartilages and nerves, when divided, will not reconstitute themselves.

29. An attack of diarrhoea puts an end to illnesses attended by the production of white phlegm.

30. The frothiness of the stools in certain cases of diarrhoea is due to substances flowing down from the head.

31. The presence of particles like coarse meal in the urine of febrile patients signifies a long illness.

32. A bilious-looking sediment in a urine which is clear above signifies an acute illness.

33. When the urine shows a deposit, there is some violent disturbance in the body.

34. Bubbles appearing on the surface of the urine indicate disease of the kidneys and a prolonged illness.

35. A considerable oily scum on the surface of the urine indicates an acute disease of the kidneys.

36. When in diseases of the kidneys the above signs occur together with acute pain in the region of the spinal muscula-

ture, an external abscess should be expected so long as the pain is felt superficially. But when the pain is located deeply, then the abscess will be situated deeply.

37. The vomiting of blood is a sign of recovery so long as it is unattended by fever; with fever it is bad. Cure may be effected in the latter case by cooling and the use of astringents.

38. Catarrh of the thoracic organs proceeds to suppuration within twenty days.

39. Patients who complain of strangury and pain in the perineum and in the pubic region, and whose urine contains blood and clots, are suffering from disease in the area round the bladder.

40. If the tongue be suddenly paralysed or if any part of the body be similarly affected, that is a sign of melancholia.

41. It is bad to purge old people so much that hiccough be produced.

42. Unless a fever be due to bile, the pouring of a lot of hot water on the head will end the fever.

43. A woman is never ambidexterous.

44. When empyemata are opened by the cautery or by the knife and the pus flows pure and white, the patient survives. But if it be mixed with blood, muddy and foul-smelling, he will die.

45. Those who are cauterized or cut for suppurating conditions of the liver survive if the pus runs pure and white, for then the abscess is encysted; if however it runs like a haemorrhage, they die.

46. Pains in the eyes should be treated by the administration of a draught of neat wine, the application of warm douches and the letting of blood.

47. There is no hope when a patient suffering from dropsy develops a cough.

48. Strangury and dysuria are relieved by the taking of neat wine and deep bleeding.

49. The appearance of redness and swelling on the chest is a good sign in cases of sore throat. It means that the disease has turned outwards.

50. Mortification of the brain is commonly followed by

death within three days, but if these be survived, recovery will follow.

51. Sneezing occurs when the brain becomes thoroughly heated or when the sinuses become thoroughly moistened or chilled. As a result the air within is pushed out and in so doing makes a noise because its exit is through a narrow passage.

52. Severe pains in the liver disappear if fever supervenes.

53. Where a patient benefits from bleeding, it is best to bleed in spring-time.

54. When phlegm is enclosed between the diaphragm and the stomach causing pain, and is then unable to burst either into the thorax or the belly, it is evacuated by the blood vessels to the bladder and so the disease is resolved.

55. When the liver is full of fluid and this overflows into the peritoneal cavity, so that the belly becomes full of water, death follows.

56. Distress, yawning and shuddering are cured by a draught of wine mixed with an equal quantity of water.

57. The pain due to tumours in the urethra is relieved when they suppurate and burst.

58. Commotion of the brain, from any cause, is inevitably followed by loss of voice.

59. A fit of choking occurring during the course of a fever where there is no swelling of the pharynx, and which results in the patient being unable to swallow except with great difficulty, is fatal.

59a. Cases of fever attended with retraction of the head and dysphagia, and yet with no swelling of the neck, are fatal.

60. Those who are suffering from oedema should be treated by starvation since starvation dries up the body.

61. Changes from hot to cold and then to hot again, affecting the whole body, or changes of colour signify a long illness.

62. Continual sweating, either hot or cold, means that there is an excess of fluid in the body. In the strong this should be removed by inducing vomiting; in the weak by purging.

63. Continued fevers are dangerous if they grow worse

every other day; should they however be remittent, in whatever fashion, it means that there is no danger.

64. Prolonged fevers are attended either by swellings or pains in the joints.

65. Those who suffer from swellings or pains of the joints as the result of fever are taking too much food.

66. If the same diet be given to a febrile patient as would be suitable for a healthy man, although it would strengthen the healthy it would cause suffering to the sick.

67. The urine must be observed to see how far it resembles that passed in health. The less it resembles healthy urine, the more diseased it is; the more it resembles it, the healthier it is.

68. Where a sediment composed, as it were, of particles forms in the stools after standing, it is necessary to give a purge. If you give gruel to the patient before having cleansed the belly you do harm and the more you give, the greater the harm.

69. Where the stools are undigested, this is due to black bile. The more pronounced this tendency, the more pronounced the disease.

70. Livid, bloody or foul-smelling sputum in cases of continued fever is bad. But if healthy sputum come away it is good. Similar principles apply to the intestines and the bladder, for when such substances remain in the body and are not evacuated it is bad.

71. Whenever it is desired to rid the body of unwanted substances, an easy evacuation is desirable. If you wish to drain the thoracic organs, you must make the bowels costive; if you wish to drain the lower organs, you must make the bowels more relaxed.

72. Sleep and wakefulness, exceeding the average, mean disease.

73. Patients of whom continued fevers have a firm hold will die if the skin is cold while the internal parts of the body are hot, and there be thirst.

74. If in the course of a continued fever a patient shows distortion of the lip, nostril or eye or if the patient, being already weak, lose his sight or his hearing, he will die.

N

75. Dropsy supervenes on white phlegm.

76. Dysentery succeeds diarrhoea.

77. Lientery succeeds dysentery.

78. A suppurative inflammation of bone succeeds caries.

79–80. The coughing up of blood is followed by consumption and the production of purulent sputum. After consumption comes a discharge from the head and after this, diarrhoea. Following diarrhoea the sputum is no longer produced and when this stops death supervenes.

81. If the urine and the stools are abnormal, or if the discharges of the flesh or any other part of the body are unusual, then a slight deviation means a slight illness, a serious disturbance a serious illness and a very serious change, death.

82. Those who contract inflammation of the brain when over forty never recover. Less risk is run by those at that age and in that state of bodily development when the disease is more usually expected.

83. If during an illness there is weeping voluntarily, it is well. But if weeping occurs in spite of oneself, it is bad.

84. Epistaxis is a bad sign in quartan fevers.

85. Fits of sweating are dangerous when they take place on days other than those of the crisis. They may be very violent, drops of sweat swiftly collecting on the forehead, and the sweat flows away from the body in cold and profuse streams. Such an attack of sweating must necessarily be attended with a violent illness, excessive pain and long-lasting distress.

86. A violent discharge from the bowels is a bad thing when it occurs during continued illness.

87. What drugs will not cure, the knife will; what the knife will not cure, the cautery will; what the cautery will not cure must be considered incurable.

THE SACRED DISEASE

An attack on the popular superstitions about epilepsy, followed by an account of the natural history of the disease.

1. I do not believe that the 'Sacred Disease' is any more divine or sacred than any other disease but, on the contrary, has specific characteristics and a definite cause. Nevertheless, because it is completely different from other diseases, it has been regarded as a divine visitation by those who, being only human, view it with ignorance and astonishment. This theory of divine origin, though supported by the difficulty of understanding the malady, is weakened by the simplicity of the cure consisting merely of ritual purification and incantation. If remarkable features in a malady were evidence of divine visitation, then there would be many 'sacred diseases'. Quotidian, tertian and quartan fevers are among other diseases no less remarkable and portentous and yet no one regards them as having a divine origin. I do not believe that these diseases have any less claim to be caused by a god than the so-called 'sacred' disease but they are not the objects of popular wonder. Again, no less remarkably, I have seen men go mad and become delirious for no obvious reason and do many strange things. I have seen many cases of people groaning and shouting in their sleep, some who choke; others jump from their bed and run outside and remain out of their mind till they wake, when they are as healthy and sane as they were before, although perhaps rather pale and weak. These things are not isolated events but frequent occurrences. There are many other remarkable afflictions of various sorts, but it would take too long to describe them in detail.

2. It is my opinion that those who first called this disease 'sacred' were the sort of people we now call witch-doctors, faith-healers, quacks and charlatans. These are exactly the people who pretend to be very pious and to be particularly wise. By invoking a divine element they were able to screen

their own failure to give suitable treatment and so called this a 'sacred' malady to conceal their ignorance of its nature. By picking their phrases carefully, prescribing purifications and incantations along with abstinence from baths and from many foods unsuitable for the sick, they ensured that their therapeutic measures were safe for themselves. The following fish were forbidden as being the most harmful: mullet, black-tail, hammer and eel. Goat, venison, pork and dog were considered most likely among meats to upset the stomach. Of fowls: cock, turtle-dove and buzzard and those which are considered very rich were forbidden; white mint, garlic and onion were excluded from the diet because over-flavoured food is not good for a sick man. Further, their patients were forbidden to wear black because it is a sign of death, to use goat-skin blankets or to wear goat-skins, nor were they allowed to put one foot on the other or one hand on the other; and all these things were regarded as preventative measures against the disease. These prohibitions are added on account of the divine element in the malady, suggesting that these practitioners had special knowledge. They also employ other pretexts so that, if the patient be cured, their reputation for cleverness is enhanced while, if he dies, they can excuse themselves by explaining that the gods are to blame while they themselves did nothing wrong; that they did not prescribe the taking of any medicine whether liquid or solid, nor any baths which might have been responsible.

I suppose none of the inhabitants of the interior of Libya can possibly be healthy seeing that they sleep on goat skins and eat goat meat. In fact, they possess neither blanket, garment nor shoe that is not made of goat skin, because goats are the only animals they keep. If contact with or eating of this animal causes the disease while abstinence from it cures the disease, then diet is alone the factor which decides the onset of the disease and its cure. No god can be blamed and the purifications are useless and the idea of divine intervention comes to nought.

3. It seems, then, that those who attempt to cure disease by this sort of treatment do not really consider the maladies thus

treated of sacred or of divine origin. If the disease can be cured
by purification and similar treatment then what is to prevent
its being brought on by like devices? The man who can get
rid of a disease by his magic could equally well bring it on;
again there is nothing divine about this but a human element
is involved. By such claims and trickery, these practitioners
pretend a deeper knowledge than is given to others; with
their prescriptions of 'sanctifications' and 'purifications', their
patter about divine visitation and possession by devils, they
seek to deceive. And yet I believe that all these professions of
piety are really more like impiety and a denial of the existence
of the gods, and all their religion and talk of divine visitation
is an impious fraud which I shall proceed to expose.

4. If these people claim to know how to draw down the
moon, cause an eclipse of the sun, make storms and fine
weather, rain and drought, to make the sea too rough for
sailing or the land infertile, and all the rest of their nonsense,
then, whether they claim to be able to do it by magic or by
some other method, they seem to be impious rogues. Either
they do not believe in the existence of the gods or they believe
that the gods are powerless or would not refrain from the most
dastardly acts. Surely conduct such as this must render them
hateful to the gods. If a man were to draw down the moon
or cause an eclipse of the sun, or make storms or fine weather
by magic and sacrifices, I should not call any of these things a
divine visitation but a human one, because the divine power
had been overcome and forced into subjection by the human
will. But perhaps these claims are not true and it is men in
search of a living who invent all these fancy tales about this
particular disease and all the others too. They make a different
god responsible for each of the different forms of the complaint.

If the sufferer acts like a goat, and if he roars, or has convulsions involving the right side, they say the Mother of the
Gods is responsible. If he utters a higher-pitched and louder
cry, they say he is like a horse and blame Poseidon. If the
sufferer should be incontinent of faeces, as sometimes happens
under the stress of an attack, Enodia is the name. If the stools

are more frequent and thin like those of kids, it is Apollo Nomius; if he foam at the mouth and kick out with his feet, Ares is to blame. If he suffers at night from fears and panic, from attacks of insanity, or if he jumps out of bed and runs outside, they talk of attacks of Hecate and the assaults of the heroes. In using purifications and spells they perform what I consider a most irreligious and impious act, for, in treating sufferers from this disease by purification with blood and like things, they behave as if the sufferers were ritually unclean, the victims of divine vengeance or of human magic or had done something sacrilegious. It would have been better if they had done the opposite and taken the sick into the temples, there, by sacrifice and prayer, to make supplication to the gods; instead they simply purify them and do none of these things. Charms are buried in the ground, thrown into the sea or carried off into the mountains where no one may touch them or tread on them. If a god really be responsible, surely these things should be taken into the temples as offerings.

Personally I believe that human bodies cannot be polluted by a god; the basest object by the most pure. But if the human body is polluted by some other agency or is harmed in some way, then the presence of a god would be more likely to purify and sanctify it than pollute it. It is the deity who purifies, sanctifies and cleanses us from the greatest and most unholy of our sins. We ourselves mark out the precincts of the temples of the gods so that no one should enter without purifying himself; as we go in, we sprinkle ourselves with holy water, not because we are thereby polluted, but to rid ourselves of any stain we may have contracted previously. This then is my opinion of the purifications.

5. I believe that this disease is not in the least more divine than any other but has the same nature as other diseases and a similar cause. Moreover, it can be cured no less than other diseases so long as it has not become inveterate and too powerful for the drugs which are given.

Like other diseases it is hereditary. If a phlegmatic child is born of a phlegmatic parent, a bilious child of a bilious parent, a consumptive child of a consumptive parent and a splenetic child of a splenetic parent, why should the children of a father or mother who is afflicted with this disease not suffer similarly? The seed comes from all parts of the body; it is healthy when it comes from healthy parts, diseased when it comes from diseased parts. Another important proof that this disease is no more divine than any other lies in the fact that the phlegmatic are constitutionally liable to it while the bilious escape. If its origin were divine, all types would be affected alike without this particular distinction.

6. So far from this being the case, the brain is the seat of this disease, as it is of other very violent diseases. I shall explain clearly the manner in which it comes about and the reason for it.

The human brain, as in the case of all other animals, is double; a thin membrane runs down the middle and divides it. This is the reason why headache is not always located in the same site but may be on either side or, sometimes, affects the whole head. There are a large number of tenuous veins which extend to this structure from all parts of the body; there are also two large vessels, one coming from the liver and one from the spleen. That which comes from the liver is disposed as follows: one half runs down on the right side in relation with the kidney and the lumbar muscles, to reach the inside of the thigh and thence continues to the foot. It is called the 'hollow vein'. The other half courses upwards through the right side of the diaphragm and lies close to the right lung; branches split off to the heart and to the right arm while the remainder passes up behind the clavicle on the right side of the neck and there lies subcutaneously so as to be visible. It disappears close to the ear and then divides; the larger part finishes in the brain while smaller branches go separately to the right ear, the right eye and to the nostril. Such is the distribution of the blood vessels from the liver. There is also a vein which extends both upwards and downwards from the spleen on the left side of the body; it is similar to that coming from the liver but is thinner and weaker.

7. It is through these blood-vessels that we respire, for they allow the body to breathe by absorbing air, and it is distributed

throughout the body by means of the minor vessels. The air is cooled in the blood-vessels and then released. Air cannot remain still but must move; if it remains still and is left behind in some part of the body, then that part becomes powerless. A proof of this is that if we compress some of the smaller blood-vessels when we are lying or sitting down, so that air cannot pass through the vessels, then numbness occurs at once. Such, then, is the nature of blood-vessels.

8. Now this disease attacks the phlegmatic but not the bilious. Its inception is even while the child is still within its mother's womb, for the brain is rid of undesirable matter and brought to full development, like the other parts, before birth. If this 'cleansing' takes place well and moderately so that neither too much nor too little comes away, the head is most healthy. But if there is too much lost from the whole brain so that a lot of wasting occurs, the head will be feeble and, when the child grows up, he will suffer from noises in the head and be unable to stand the sun or the cold. If the discharge is excessive from one part only, such as an eye or an ear, or one blood-vessel becomes shrivelled up, then whichever part be wasted in that way becomes damaged. On the other hand, if this 'cleansing' does not take place but the material is retained in the brain, a phlegmatic constitution is bound to result.

Sometimes phlegm, which should have been purged out during life in the womb, remains during early life and is only got rid of in the later years. This is what happens in the case of children who suffer from ulcers of the head, ears and flesh, and who salivate and discharge mucus; they get better as they grow older. Those who have been purged of the phlegm in this way are not troubled by this disease, but for those who have neither been purged in this way by ulceration and discharges of mucus and saliva, nor have been purged in the womb, it is most dangerous to be attacked with it.

9. If these discharges should make their way to the heart, the chest is attacked and palpitation or asthma supervenes; some patients even become kyphotic. For when cold mucus reaches the lungs and heart, the blood is chilled and the blood-vessels, as a result of being violently cooled in the region of

the lungs and heart, jump and the heart palpitates. Such circumstances force the onset of asthma and diseases characterized by orthopnoea because, until the mucus which has flowed down has been warmed and dissipated by the blood-vessels, it is impossible to inspire as much air as is needed. When the phlegm has been removed, palpitation and asthma stop. The length of an attack depends upon the quantity of mucus which has flowed in. The more frequent these discharges of mucus, the more frequent the attacks. These effects, however, occur only if the discharge makes its way to the lungs and heart; if it reaches the stomach, diarrhoea results.

10. Should these routes for the passage of phlegm from the brain be blocked, the discharge enters the blood vessels which I have described. This causes aphonia, choking, foaming at the mouth, clenching of the teeth and convulsive movements of the hands; the eyes are fixed, the patient becomes unconscious and, in some cases, passes a stool. I will explain the reason for each of these signs. Loss of voice occurs when the phlegm suddenly descends in the blood-vessels and blocks them so that air can pass neither to the brain nor to the hollow blood-vessels nor to the body cavities, and thereby inhibits respiration. For when a man draws in breath through the mouth and nose, the air passes first to the brain and then the greater part goes to the stomach, but some flows into the lungs and blood-vessels. From these places it is dispensed throughout the rest of the body by means of the blood-vessels. The air which flows into the stomach cools it but makes no other contribution. But that which goes to the lungs and blood-vessels thence enters the body cavities and the brain and has a further purpose. It induces intelligence and is necessary for the movement of the limbs. Therefore, when the blood-vessels are shut off from this supply of air by the accumulation of phlegm and thus cannot afford it passage, the patient loses his voice and his wits. The hands become powerless and move convulsively for the blood can no longer maintain its customary flow. Divergence of the eyes takes place when the smaller blood-vessels supplying them are shut off and no

longer provide an air supply; the vessels then pulsate. The froth which appears at the lips comes from the lungs for, when air no longer enters them, they produce froth which is expectorated as in the dying. The violence of choking causes the passage of stools; choking is caused by the liver and the thoracic contents compressing the diaphragm and thus obstructing the entry into the stomach. This action results from the amount of air taken in by the mouth being less than normal. When air is shut off in the vessels of the limbs and cannot escape owing to the obstruction of the vessels with phlegm, it moves violently up and down through the blood and the convulsions and pain thus caused produce the kicking movements.

All these symptoms are produced when cold phlegm is discharged into the blood which is warm, so chilling the blood and obstructing its flow. If the cold material is copious and thick, the result is immediately fatal as though its coldness had overcome and destroyed the blood. If the quantity is less, however, although at first it may have the upper hand and obstruct respiration, in the end it is dispersed throughout the blood which is plentiful and warm, and if it be overcome in this way, the blood-vessels again take in air and consciousness returns.

11. Infants who suffer from this disease usually die if the phlegm is copious and if the weather is southerly. Their little blood-vessels are too narrow to absorb a large quantity of inspissated phlegm and so the blood is at once chilled and frozen, thus causing death. If the amount of phlegm is small and enters both main vessels, or if it enters but one of them, the patient survives but bears the stigmata. Thus the mouth may be distorted, or an eye, a hand or the neck; according to the part of the body in which some blood-vessel became filled and obstructed with phelgm and thus rendered inadequate. As a result of this damage to the blood-vessel, the corresponding part of the body must necessarily be weakened.

Taking a long view such a happening is generally a good thing because a child is not liable to another attack after an attack which has produced some permanent damage. The reason for this is that the strain of the attack causes injury to and some narrowing of the remaining blood-vessels. As a result of this they will no longer admit the entry of phlegm to the same extent although they will admit air. It is, however, only to be expected that such deterioration in the condition of the blood-vessels will lead to some weakening of the limbs.

Those who have a very small discharge at a time when the weather is northerly recover without any permanent injury, but there is a danger in such cases that the disease will remain with the child as he grows older.

Such, then, is the way in which, more or less, this malady affects children.

12. Adults neither die from an attack of this disease, nor does it leave them with palsy. The blood-vessels in patients of this age are capacious and full of hot blood; as a result, the phlegm cannot gain the upper hand and chill and freeze the blood. Instead the phlegm is quickly overcome as it is diluted by the blood, and the vessels take in air again so that consciousness returns and the symptoms mentioned above are less pronounced owing to the strength of the patient.

Attacks of this disease in the aged are not fatal, nor do they cause paralysis. The reason is that the vessels are empty and the blood small in quantity and of thin and watery consistency. Nevertheless, a severe discharge of phlegm in winter may prove fatal if it takes place on both sides of the body by obstructing respiration and congealing the blood. If the discharge takes place on one side only, then, because the blood is too little, too cold and too thin, it cannot overcome the phlegm but instead is itself overcome and frozen. As a result, those parts of the body where the blood is destroyed become powerless.

13. The discharge of phlegm takes place more often on the right side of the body than on the left because the blood-vessels on that side are more numerous and of greater calibre than on the left.

The liquefaction and the subsequent discharge of phlegm occurs specially in children whose heads have been warmed thoroughly either by the sun or at a fire, and have then had the brain suddenly cooled, thus producing a separation of the phlegm. Although liquefying is produced by warmth and relaxation of the brain, it is the chilling and consolidating which makes the phlegm separate out, and thus causes the discharge. Such is the explanation in some cases; in others, after a period in which the wind has been in the North for some time and then shifts to the South, the brain which is consolidated and healthy becomes soft and relaxed. A discharge may also occur from obscure causes as when a patient has a fright, or is startled by someone shouting, or when sobs will not let him take in a breath quickly enough, as often happens with children. When such things happen the body immediately becomes cold and aphonia is succeeded by apnoea. When breathing stops the brain congeals and the blood stops; thus the phlegm is secreted and discharged. Such are the causes of fits from which children at first may suffer.

In older people, the winter is the most dangerous time. When they get their heads and brains warm in front of a roaring fire and then go out and shiver in the cold, or when they come out of the cold into a warm room and a hot fire, the same thing happens for the reasons already given and they have a fit. There is also a grave risk of the same thing happening in the spring as a result of sun-stroke; it is least likely to happen in the summer when there are no sudden variations in temperature. Cases who have been free from the disease in childhood having their first attack after the age of twenty, are very rare if not unheard of. At this time of life the vessels are filled with a great quantity of blood while the brain is stiff and solid. There is thus no discharge into the blood vessels or, if there is, it does not overcome the blood because this is so ample and warm.

14. When the disease has been present from childhood, a habit develops of attacks occurring at any change of wind and specially when it is southerly. This is hard to cure because the brain has become more moist than normal and is flooded with phlegm. This renders discharges more frequent. The phlegm can no longer be completely separated out; neither can the brain, which remains wet and soaked, be dried up.

This observation results specially from a study of animals, particularly of goats which are liable to this disease. Indeed, they are peculiarly susceptible to it. If you cut open the head you will find that the brain is wet, full of fluid and foul-smelling, convincing proof that disease and not the deity is harming the body. It is just the same with man, for when the malady becomes chronic, it becomes incurable. The brain is dissolved by phlegm and liquefies; the melted substance thus formed turns into water which surrounds the brain on the outside and washes round it like the sea round an island. Consequently, fits become more frequent and require less to cause them. The disease therefore becomes very chronic as the fluid surrounding the brain is dilute because its quantity is so great, and as a result it may be quickly overcome by the blood and warmed.

15. Patients who suffer from this disease have a premonitory indication of an attack. In such circumstances they avoid company, going home if they are near enough, or to the loneliest spot they can find if they are not, so that as few people as possible will see them fall, and they at once wrap their heads up in their coats. This is the normal reaction to embarrassment and not, as most people suppose, from fear of the demon. Small children, from inexperience and being unaccustomed to the disease, at first fall down wherever they happen to be. Later, after a number of attacks, they run to their mothers or to someone whom they know well when they feel one coming on. This is through fear and fright at what they feel, for they have not yet learnt to feel ashamed.

16. The reasons for attacks occurring when there is a change of wind are, I believe, the following. Attacks are most likely to occur when the wind is southerly; less when it is northerly, less still when it is in any other quarter; for the South and North winds are the strongest of the winds and the most opposed in direction and in influence. The North wind precipitates the moisture in the air so that the cloudy and damp elements are separated out leaving the atmosphere clear and bright. It treats similarly all the other vapours which arise from the sea or from other stretches of water, distilling out

from them the damp and dark elements. It does the same for human beings and it is therefore the healthiest wind. The South wind has just the opposite effect. It starts by vaporizing the precipitated moisture because it does not generally blow very hard at first. This calm period occurs because the wind cannot immediately absorb the moisture in the air which was previously dense and congealed, but loosens it in time. The South wind has the same effect on the earth, the sea, rivers, springs, wells and everything that grows or contains moisture. In fact, everything contains moisture in a greater or lesser degree and thus all these things feel the effect of the South wind and become dark instead of bright, warm instead of cold and moist instead of dry. Jars in the house or in the cellars which contain wine or any other liquid are influenced by the South wind and change their shape. The South wind also makes the sun, moon and stars much dimmer than usual.

Seeing that such large and powerful bodies are overcome and that the human body is made to feel changes of wind and undergo changes at that time, it follows that southerly winds relax the brain and make it flabby, relaxing the blood-vessels at the same time. Northerly winds, on the other hand, solidify the healthy part of the brain while any morbid part is separated out and forms a fluid layer round the outside. Thus it is that discharges occur when the wind changes. It is seen, then, that this disease rises and flourishes according to changes we can see come and go. It is no more difficult to understand, nor is it any more divine than any other malady.

17. It ought to be generally known that the source of our pleasure, merriment, laughter and amusement, as of our grief, pain, anxiety and tears, is none other than the brain. It is specially the organ which enables us to think, see and hear, and to distinguish the ugly and the beautiful, the bad and the good, pleasant and unpleasant. Sometimes we judge according to convention; at other times according to the perceptions of expediency. It is the brain too which is the seat of madness and delirium, of the fears and frights which assail us, often by night, but sometimes even by day; it is there where lies the cause of insomnia and sleep-walking, of thoughts that will not

come, forgotten duties and eccentricities. All such things result from an unhealthy condition of the brain; it may be warmer than it should be, or it may be colder, or moister or drier, or in any other abnormal state. Moistness is the cause of madness for when the brain is abnormally moist it is necessarily agitated and this agitation prevents sight or hearing being steady. Because of this, varying visual and acoustic sensations are produced, while the tongue can only describe things as they appear and sound. So long as the brain is still, a man is in his right mind.

18. The brain may be attacked both by phlegm and by bile and the two types of disorder which result may be distinguished thus: those whose madness results from phlegm are quiet and neither shout nor make a disturbance; those whose madness results from bile shout, play tricks and will not keep still but are always up to some mischief. Such are the causes of continued madness, but fears and frights may be caused by changes in the brain. Such a change occurs when it is warmed and that is the effect bile has when, flowing from the rest of the body, it courses to the brain along the blood-vessels. Fright continues until the bile runs away again into the blood-vessels and into the body. Feelings of pain and nausea result from inopportune cooling and abnormal consolidation of the brain and this is the effect of phlegm. The same condition is responsible for loss of memory. Those of a bilious constitution are liable to shout and to cry out during the night when the brain is suddenly heated; those of phlegmatic constitution do not suffer in this way. Warming of the brain also takes place when a plethora of blood finds its way to the brain and boils. It courses along the blood-vessels I have described in great quantity when a man is having a nightmare and is in a state of terror. He reacts in sleep in the same way that he would if he were awake; his face burns, his eyes are blood-shot as they are when scared or when the mind is intent upon the commission of a crime. All this ceases as soon as the man wakes and the blood is dispersed again into the blood vessels.

19. For these reasons I believe the brain to be the most potent organ in the body. So long as it is healthy, it is the

interpreter which enables us to draw anything from the air. Consciousness is caused by air. The eyes, ears, tongue, hands and feet perform actions which are planned by the brain, for there is a measure of conscious thought throughout the body proportionate to the amount of air which it receives. The brain is also the organ of comprehension, for when a man draws in a breath it reaches the brain first, and thence is dispersed into the rest of the body having left behind in the brain its vigour and whatever pertains to consciousness and intelligence. If the air went first to the body and subsequently to the brain, the power of understanding would be left to the flesh and to the blood-vessels; it would only reach the brain hot and when it was no longer pure owing to admixture with fluid from the tissues and from the blood and this would blunt its keenness.

20. I therefore assert that the brain is the interpreter of comprehension. Accident and convention have falsely ascribed that function to the diaphragm[1] which does not and could not possess it. I know of no way in which the diaphragm can think and be conscious, except that a sudden access of pleasure or of pain might make it jump and throb because it is so thin and is under greater tension than any other part of the body. Moreover, it has no cavity into which it might receive anything good or bad that comes upon it, but the weakness of its construction makes it liable to disturbance by either of these forces. It is no quicker in perception than any other part of the body, and its name and associations are quite unwarranted, just as parts of the heart are called auricles though they make no contribution to hearing. Some say too that we think with our hearts and it is the heart which suffers pain and feels anxiety. There is no truth in this although it is convulsed as is the diaphragm and even more for the following reasons: blood-vessels from all parts of the body run to the heart and these connections ensure that it can feel if any pain or strain occurs in the body. Moreover, the body cannot help giving a shudder and a contraction when subjected to pain and the same effect

---

[1] Gk. *phrenes* (diaphragm) is frequently used for 'mind' in the widest sense. The words for thinking, consciousness, etc., are closely connected.

is produced by an excess of joy, which heart and diaphragm feel most intensely. Neither of these organs takes any part in mental operations which are completely undertaken by the brain. As then the brain is the first organ in the body to perceive the consciousness derived from the air, if the seasons cause any violent change in the air, the brain undergoes its greatest variations. This is my reason for asserting that the diseases which attack the brain are the most acute, most serious and most fatal, and the hardest problem in diagnosis for the unskilled practitioner.

21. This so-called 'sacred disease' is due to the same causes as all other diseases, to the things we see come and go, the cold and the sun too, the changing and inconstant winds. These things are divine so that there is no need to regard this disease as more divine than any other; all are alike divine and all human. Each has its own nature and character and there is nothing in any disease which is unintelligible or which is insusceptible to treatment. The majority of maladies may be cured by the same things as caused them. One thing nourishes one thing, another another and sometimes destroys it too. The physician must know of these things in order to be able to recognize the opportune moment to nourish and increase one thing while robbing another of its sustinence and so destroy it.

In this disease as in all others, it should be your aim to wear it down by applying the remedies most hostile to the disease and those things to which it is unaccustomed. A malady flourishes and grows in its accustomed circumstances but is blunted and declines when attacked by a hostile sub- stance. A man with the knowledge of how to produce by means of a regimen dryness and moisture, cold and heat in the human body, could cure this disease too provided that he could distinguish the right moment for the application of the remedies. He would not need to resort to purifications and magic spells.

O

DREAMS

This short treatise on the medical significance of dreams forms the conclusion to a long work on Regimen; *this explains the numbering of the paragraphs, and the last sentence must be understood to refer to the whole work.*

86. Accurate knowledge about the signs which occur in dreams will be found very valuable for all purposes. While the body is awake, the psyche is not under its own control, but is split into various portions each being devoted to some special bodily function such as hearing, vision, touch, locomotion and all the various actions of the body. But when the body is at rest, the psyche is stirred and roused and becomes its own master; the mind itself performs all the functions of the body. When the body is sleeping it receives no sensations, but the psyche being awake at that time perceives everything; it sees what is visible, it hears what is audible, it walks, it touches, it feels pain and thinks. In short, during sleep the psyche performs all the functions of both body and mind. A correct appreciation of these things implies considerable wisdom.

87. There are special interpreters, with their own science of these matters, for the god-given dreams which give to cities or to individuals foreknowledge of the future. Such people also interpret the signs derived from the psyche which indicate bodily states; excess or lack of what is natural, or of some unusual change. In such matters they are sometimes right and sometimes wrong, but in neither case do they know why it happens, whether they are right or wrong, but nevertheless they give advice so you shall 'beware of taking harm'. Yet they never show you how you ought to beware, but merely tell you to pray to the gods. Prayer is a good thing, but one should take on part of the burden oneself and call on the gods only to help.

88. The facts about dreams are as follows: those that merely consist of a transference to the night of a person's daytime actions and thoughts, which continue to happen in normal fashion just as they were done and thought during the day, are good for they indicate a healthy state. This is because the psyche remains true to its daytime cogitations, and is overcome neither by excess nor by emptiness, nor by any other extraneous circumstance. But when dreams take on a character contrary to daytime activity and involve conflict or victory over them, then they constitute a sign of bodily disturbance. The seriousness of the conflict is an indication of the seriousness of the mischief. Now concerning this, I make no judgement whether or not you ought to avert the consequence by appropriate rites or not. But I do advise treatment of the body, for an excretion resulting from some bodily superfluity has disturbed the psyche. If the opposing force be strong, it is a good thing to give an emetic and to administer a gradually increasing light diet for five days, to order frequent early-morning walks gradually becoming more brisk, and gymnastics for those accustomed to this form of exercise, proportionate in severity to the increase of diet. If the opposing force be weaker, dispense with the emetic, reduce the diet by a third and restore the cut by a gradual measure over five days. Strenuous walks and the use of vocal exercises will put an end to the disturbance.

89. It is a good sign to see the sun, moon, sky and stars clear and undimmed, each being placed normally in its right place, since it shows that the body is well and free from disturbing influences. But it is necessary to follow a régime which will ensure that such a condition is maintained. On the contrary, if any of these celestial bodies appear displaced or changed then such a sign indicates bodily disease, the severity of which depends upon the seriousness of the interference.

Now the orbit of the stars is the outermost, that of the sun is intermediate, while that of the moon is nearest to the hollow vault of the sky. Should one of the stars seem to be injured, or should it disappear or stop in its revolution as a result of mist or cloud, this is a weak sign. If such a change be produced by rain or hail, it is stronger and signifies that an excretion of moisture and phlegm has occurred into the corresponding outermost parts. In such cases, prescribe long runs well wrapped up, increasing the exercise so as to cause as much sweating as possible. The exercise should be followed by long walks and the patient should go without breakfast. Food should be cut by a third and the normal diet restored gradually over five days. If the disorder appears more severe, prescribe vapour baths in addition. It is advisable to cleanse through the skin because the harm is in the outermost parts. Therefore prescribe dry, pungent, bitter, undiluted foods and the most dehydrating exercises.

If the moon is involved, it is advisable to draw off the harmful matter internally; therefore to use an emetic following the administration of pungent, salty and soft foods. Also, prescribe brisk runs on a circular track, walks and vocal exercises. Forbid breakfast and reduce the food intake, restoring it as before. The cleansing should be done internally because the harm appeared in the hollows of the body.

If the sun encounters any of these changes, the trouble is more violent and less easy to expel. The drawing-off should be produced both ways; prescribe runs on the stadium track and on the circular track, walks and all other forms of exercise. Give an emetic, cut the food and restore the diet gradually over five days as before.

If the heavenly bodies are seen dimly in a clear sky, and shine weakly and seem to be stopped from revolving by dryness, then it is a sign that there is a danger of incurring sickness. Exercise should be stopped while a fluid diet, frequent baths and plenty of rest and sleep should be prescribed until there is a return to normal.

If the heavenly bodies are opposed by a fiery atmosphere, the excretion of bile is indicated. If the opposing powers get the upper hand, sickness is portended; but if they completely overcome the stars and these vanish, then there is danger that the sickness may terminate fatally. If the opposing influences, however, are put to flight and it seems as if they are pursued by the heavenly bodies, then there is danger of the patient going mad unless he be treated. In all these cases, it is best to start treatment by purging with hellebore. If this is not done, the diet should be fluid and no wine should be taken unless it be white and well-diluted. Warm, pungent, dehydrating and salt things should be avoided. Prescribe as much natural exercise as possible and plenty of runs with the patients well wrapped-up. Avoid massage, wrestling and wrestling in dust. Soften them with plenty of sleep and, apart from natural exercise, let them rest. Let them take a walk after dinner. It is also good to take a vapour bath followed by an emetic. For thirty days the patient should not eat his fill, but when he is restored to a full diet he should take an emetic thrice monthly after partaking of a sweet, fluid and light meal.

When the heavenly bodies wander in different directions, some mental disturbance as a result of anxiety is indicated. In this case, ease is beneficial. The mind should be turned to entertainments, especially amusing ones, or failing these, any that may give special pleasure, for two or three days. This may effect a cure; if not, the mental anxiety may engender disease.

It is a sign of health if a star, which is clear and bright, appears to fall out of its orbit and to move eastwards. The separation of any clear substance and its natural excretion from the body is good. Thus excretion of substances into the bowels and the formation of abscessions in the skin are examples of things falling out of their orbit.

It is a sign of sickness if the star appears dim and moves either westward, or down into the earth or sea, or upwards. Upward movement indicates fluxes in the head; movement into the sea, disease of the bowels; earthward movement, the growing of tumours in the flesh. In these cases it is wise to reduce the food intake by a third and, after an emetic, to increase it over five days. Then a normal diet should be taken for a further five days, after which another emetic should be taken followed by an increase in the same way.

It is a healthy sign if any of the heavenly bodies appears clear and moist, because the influx from the ether acting on the person is clear and the mind perceives this as it enters. If it be dark and obscure, then sickness is indicated, not due to some internal excess or lack of something, but coming from the external environment. In this case it is advisable to take brisk runs on a circular track so as to restrict the wasting of the body. Also, the quickened respiration causes excretion of the intruding influence, and brisk walks should follow the runs. The diet should be soft and light, being increased to reach the normal in four days.

When a person appears to receive something pure from a pure deity, it is good for health because it means that the things entering his body are pure. If he seems to see the opposite of this, it is not good because it indicates that some element of disease has entered his body. Such a case should be treated as the one described above.

If it seems to rain with gentle rain from clear skies, and without any violent downpour or heavy storm, it is good. Such indicates that the breath drawn from the air is proportionate and pure. If the reverse happens, violent rain, storm and tempest, and the rain is not clear, it indicates the onset of disease from the respired air. A similar régime should be prescribed for this sort of case and very little food should be taken.

From the information which comes from this knowledge of the heavenly bodies, one must take precautions and follow the prescribed regimens. Pray to the gods: when the signs are good to the Sun, to Zeus of the sky, Zeus of the home, Athena of the home, to Hermes and Apollo. When the signs are the opposite, pray to the gods who avert evil, to Earth and to the Heroes, that all ills may be turned aside.

90. The following are some of the signs that foretell health; to see clearly and to hear distinctly things on the earth, to walk safely and to run safely and swiftly without fear, to see the earth smooth and well tilled and trees flourishing, laden with fruit and well-kept; to see rivers flowing normally with water clear and neither in flood nor with their flow lessened, and springs and wells similarly. All these things indicate the subject's health, and that the body, its circulation, the food ingested and the excreta, are normal.

Anything seen which is the contrary, however, indicates

something wrong in the body. Interference with sight or hearing indicates some malady of the head and longer early morning and after dinner walks than in the previous regimen should be ordered. If the legs are harmed, a contrary pull should be exerted by emetics and a greater indulgence in wrestling. Rough land indicates impurity in the flesh; longer walks after exercise should be ordered.

Trees that do not bear fruit indicate destruction of the human semen; if the trees are losing their leaves the cause of the trouble is wet and cold; if they are flourishing but barren, heat and dryness. In the one case, the regimen should aim at warming and drying; in the other, at cooling and moistening.

Abnormality in rivers relates to the circulation of the blood. If the flow be greater than usual, a superfluity of blood; if it be less, a deficiency. The regimen should aim at a decrease or an increase respectively. If the water is cloudy, some disturbance is indicated. This can be remedied by runs on a track or by walking; increased breathing disperses it.

Springs and wells relate to the bladder and in these cases diuretics should be employed.

A rough sea indicates disease of the bowels. Light and gentle laxatives should be used to effect a thorough purgation.

An earth-tremor or the shaking of a house predicts the onset of sickness when it is observed by a healthy man; a change and the restoration of health for a sick one. In the healthy, it is wise to change the regimen because it is the existing régime which is disturbing the whole body; therefore first give an emetic so that, after this, he may be fed up again gradually. But in the case of a sick man, because the body itself is undergoing a change, the same regimen should be continued.

To see land flooded with water or by the sea is a sign of illness, indicating excess fluid in the body. Prescribe emetics, fasting, exercise and a dry diet increasing little by little. Nor is it good to see the earth looking black or scorched; this shows excessive dehydration of the body and there is the risk of severe or fatal illness. Stop exercise and forbid all dry, pungent and diuretic food. Prescribe boiled barley-water and a small quantity of light food together with plenty of watery white wine to drink and lots of baths. The patient should not bath till he has eaten; then let him lie soft and relax, avoiding cold and sun. Pray to Earth, Hermes and the Heroes. To dream of diving into a lake, the sea or rivers is not a good sign as it too indicates an excess of moisture. It is advisable to use a dehydrating regimen and more exercise. In those suffering from fever, however, it is a good sign, indicating that the heat is being quenched by moisture.

91. It is a good sign for health to see anything normal about one's clothing, the size being neither too large nor too small but in accordance with one's own size. It is good to have white garments of one's own and the finest footwear. Anything too large or too small for one's limbs is not good; in the one case the regimen should aim at a decrease, and in the other, an increase. Black things indicate a more sickly or dangerous condition. Softening and moistening measures should be applied. New things denote a change.

92. To see the dead, clean, in white clothes, is good; while to receive something clean from them denotes health both of body and mind. This is because the dead are a source of nourishment, increase and propagation, and it is a sign of health that these should enter the body clean. On the contrary, if the dead appear naked, or in dark garments, or unclean, or taking or carrying anything out of the house, this is an inexpedient sign indicating disease because the things entering the body are harmful. These should be purged away by circular runs and walks and, after an emetic, a soft and light diet should be given which is gradually increased.

93. The appearance of monstrous creatures which appear during sleep and frighten the dreamer indicate a surfeit or unaccustomed food, a secretion, cholera and a dangerous illness. An emetic should be followed by an increasing diet of the lightest foods for five days; the food should neither be excessive nor pungent, nor dry nor warm. Prescribe also exercise, especially natural exercise, but not walks after dinner. Warm baths and relaxation are also advisable, and both the sun and the cold should be avoided.

To seem, while sleeping, to eat or to drink one's normal diet indicates undernourishment and a mental hunger. The stronger the meats seem, the greater the degree of inadequacy of the diet; weaker meats indicate a smaller deficiency, as if it were good to partake of whatever were seen in the dream. . . .[1] The diet should therefore be reduced, as it indicates a surfeit of nourishment. To dream of loaves made with cheese and honey has a similar significance.

Drinking clear water is not harmful; all other sorts of water are. Any normal things seen in a dream indicate a similar appetite of the mind.

If the dreamer flies in fright from anything, this means a failure of the circulation as a result of dehydration. It is then wise to cool and moisten the body.

Fighting, being stabbed or bound by another indicates that some secretion, inimical to the circulation, has taken place into the body. It is then advisable to take an emetic, to go on a reducing diet and to go for walks. A light diet, increasing over four days, should be taken after the emetic. Wandering and difficult climbs have the same meaning.

Fording rivers, enemy soldiers and monstrous apparitions denote illness or madness. After an emetic give a small diet of light soft food, increasing gently for five days, together with plenty of exercise except walks after dinner, warm baths and relaxation. Avoid cold and sun.

By following the instructions I have given, one may live a healthy life; and I have discovered the best regimen that can be devised by a mere mortal with the help of the gods.

[1] A sentence is probably lost here.

THE NATURE OF MAN

A popular lecture on physiology.

1. This lecture is not intended for those who are accustomed to hear discourses which inquire more deeply into the human constitution than is profitable for medical study. I am not going to assert that man is all air, or fire, or water, or earth, or in fact anything but what manifestly composes his body; let those who like discuss such matters. Nevertheless, when these things are discussed I perceive a certain discrepancy in the analyses for, although the same theory is employed, the conclusions do not agree. They all, theorizing, draw the same deduction, asserting that there is one basic substance which is unique and the basis of everything; but they call it by different names, one insisting that it is air, another that it is fire, another water, another earth. Each adds arguments and proofs to support his contention, all of which mean nothing. Now, whenever people arguing on the same theory do not reach the same conclusion, you may be sure that they do not know what they are talking about. A good illustration of this is provided by attending their disputations when the same disputants are present and the same audience; the same man never wins the argument three times running, it is first one and then the other and sometimes the one who happens to have the glibbest tongue. Yet it would be expected that the man who asserts that he can provide the correct explanation of the subject, if, that is, he really knows what he is talking about and demonstrates it correctly, should always win the argument. I am of the opinion that these people wreck their own theories on the problem of terminology because they fail to understand the issue. Thus they serve, rather, to establish the theory of Melissus.[1]

2. I need say no more about these theorists. But when we

[1] Flourished about 440 B.C.; he denied the possibility of complete human knowledge.

come to physicians, we find that some assert that man is composed of blood, others of bile and some of phlegm. But these, too, all make the same point asserting that there is a basic unity of substance, although they each give it a different name and so change its appearance and properties under stress of heat and cold, becoming sweet or bitter, white or black, and so forth. Now I do not agree with these people either, although the majority will declare that this, or something very similar, is the case. I hold that if man were basically of one substance, he would never feel pain, since, being one, there would be nothing to hurt. Moreover, if he should feel pain, the remedy likewise would have to be single. But in fact there are many remedies because there are many things in the body which when abnormally heated, cooled, dried or moistened by interaction, engender disease. As a result, disease has a plurality of forms and a plurality of cures.

I challenge the man who asserts that blood is the sole constituent of the human body, to show, not that it undergoes changes into all sorts of forms, but that there is a time of year or of human life when blood is obviously the sole constituent of the body. It is reasonable to suppose, were this theory true, that there is one period at which it appears in its proper form. The same applies to those who make the body of phlegm or bile.

I propose to show that the substances I believe compose the body are, both nominally and essentially, always the same and unchanging; in youth as well as in age, in cold weather as well as in warm. I shall produce proofs and demonstrate the causes both of the growth and decline of each of the constituents of the body.

3. In the first place, generation cannot arise from a single substance. For how could one thing generate another unless it copulated with some other? Secondly, unless the things which copulated were of the same species and had the same generative capabilities, we should not get these results. Again, generation would be impossible unless the hot stood in a fair and reasonable proportion to the cold, and likewise the dry to the wet; if, for instance, one preponderated over the other,

one being much stronger and the other much weaker. Is it likely, then, that anything should be generated from one thing, seeing that not even a number of things suffice unless they are combined in the right proportions? It follows, then, such being the nature of the human body and of everything else, that man is not a unity but each of the elements contributing to his formation preserves in the body the potentiality which it contributed. It also follows that each of the elements must return to its original nature when the body dies; the wet to the wet, the dry to the dry, the hot to the hot and the cold to the cold. The constitution of animals is similar and of everything else too. All things have a similar generation and a similar dissolution, for all are formed of the substances mentioned and are finally resolved in the same constituents as produced them; that too is how they disappear.

4. The human body contains blood, phlegm, yellow bile and black bile. These are the things that make up its constitution and cause its pains and health. Health is primarily that state in which these constituent substances are in the correct proportion to each other, both in strength and quantity, and are well mixed. Pain occurs when one of the substances presents either a deficiency or an excess, or is separated in the body and not mixed with the others. It is inevitable that when one of these is separated from the rest and stands by itself, not only the part from which it has come, but also that where it collects and is present in excess, should become diseased, and because it contains too much of the particular substance, cause pain and distress. Whenever there is more than slight discharge of one of these humours outside the body, then its loss is accompanied by pain. If, however, the loss, change or separation from the other humours is internal, then it inevitably causes twice as much pain, as I have said, for pain is produced both in the part whence it is derived and in the part where it accumulates.

5. Now I said that I would demonstrate that my proposed constituents of the human body were always constant, both nominally and essentially. I hold that these constituents are

blood, phlegm and yellow and black bile. They have specific
and different names because there are essential differences in
their appearance. Phlegm is not like blood, nor is blood like
bile, nor bile like phlegm. Indeed, how could they be alike
when there is no similarity in appearance and when they are
different to the sense of touch. They are dissimilar in their
qualities of heat, cold, dryness and moisture. It follows then
that substances so unlike in appearance and characteristics
cannot basically be identical, at least if fire and water are not
identical. As evidence of the fact that they are dissimilar, each
possessing its own qualities and nature, consider the following
case. If you give a man medicine which brings up phlegm, you
will find his vomit is phlegm; if you give him one which
brings up bile, he will vomit bile. Similarly, black bile can be
eliminated by administering a medicine which brings it up, or,
if you cut the body so as to form an open wound, it bleeds.
These things will take place just the same every day and every
night, winter and summer, so long as the subject can draw
breath and expel it again, or until he is deprived of any of
these congenital elements. For they must be congenital, firstly
because it is obvious that they are present at every age so long
as life is present and, secondly, because they were procreated
by a human being who had them all and mothered in a human
being similarly endowed with all the elements which I have
indicated and demonstrated.

6. Those who assert that the human body is a single substance seem to have reasoned along the following lines.
Having observed that when men died from excessive purgation following the administration of drugs, some vomited bile
and some phlegm, they concluded from this that whatever
was the nature of the material voided at death, this was indeed
the fundamental constituent of man. Those who insist that
blood is the basic substance use a similar argument; because
they see blood flowing from the body in the fatally wounded,
they conclude that blood constitutes the soul. They all use
similar arguments to support their theories. But, to begin
with, no one ever yet died from excessive purgation and
brought up only bile; taking medicine which causes the

bringing up of bile, produces first the vomiting of bile, but subsequently, the vomiting of phlegm as well. This is followed by the vomiting of black bile in spite of themselves and they end up by vomiting pure blood and that is how they die. The same effects result from taking a drug which brings up phlegm; the vomiting of phlegm is followed by yellow bile, then black bile, then pure blood, and so death ensues. When a drug is ingested, it first causes the evacuation of whatever in the body is naturally suited to it, but afterwards, it causes the voiding of other substances too. It is similar in the case of plants and seeds; when these are put into the ground, they first absorb the things which naturally suit them; they may be acid, bitter, sweet, salty and so forth. But although at first the plant takes what is naturally suited to it, afterwards it absorbs other things as well. The action of drugs in the body is similar; those which cause the bringing up of bile at first bring it up undiluted, but later on it is voided mixed with other substances; the same is true of drugs which bring up phlegm. In the case of men who have been fatally wounded the blood at first runs very warm and red, but subsequently it becomes more like phlegm and bile.

7. Now the quantity of phlegm in the body increases in winter because it is that bodily substance most in keeping with the winter, seeing that it is the coldest. You can verify its coldness by touching phlegm, bile and blood; you will find that the phlegm is the coldest. It is however the most viscous and is brought up with greater force than any other substance with the exception of black bile. Although those things which are forcibly expelled become warmer owing to the force to which they are subjected, nevertheless phlegm remains the coldest substance, and obviously so, owing to its natural characteristics. The following signs show that winter fills the body with phlegm: people spit and blow from their noses the most phlegmatic mucus in winter; swellings become white especially at that season and other diseases show phlegmatic signs.

During the spring, although the phlegm remains strong in the body, the quantity of blood increases. Then, as the cold becomes less intense and the rainy season comes on, the wet and warm days increase further the quantity of blood. This part of the year is most in keeping with blood because it is wet and hot. That this is so, you can judge by these signs: it is in spring and summer that people are particularly liable to dysentery and to epistaxis, and these are the seasons too at which people are warmest and their complexions are ruddiest.

During the summer, the blood is still strong but the bile gradually increases, and this change continues into the autumn when the blood decreases since the autumn is contrary to it. The bile rules the body during the summer and the autumn. As proof of this, it is during this season that people vomit bile spontaneously, or, if they take drugs, they void the most bilious sort of matter. It is plain too from the nature of fevers and from people's complexions in that season. During the summer, the phlegm is at its weakest since this season, on account of its dryness and heat, is most contrary to that substance.

The blood in the body reaches its lowest level in autumn, because this is a dry season and the body is already beginning to cool. Black bile is strongest and preponderates in the autumn. When winter sets in the bile is cooled and decreases while the phlegm increases again owing to the amount of rain and the length of the nights.

All these substances, then, are all always present in the body but vary in their relative quantities, each preponderating in turn according to its natural characteristics. The year has its share of all the elements; heat, cold, dryness and wetness. None of these could exist alone, while, on the other hand, were they missing, all would disappear, for they are all mutually inter-dependent. In the same way, if any of these primary bodily substances were absent, life would cease. And just as the year is governed at one time by winter, then by spring, then by summer and then by autumn; so at one time in the body phlegm preponderates, at another time blood, at another time yellow bile and this is followed by the preponderance of black bile. A very clear proof of this can be obtained by giving the same man the same emetic at four different times in the year; his vomit will be most phlegmatic in winter, most wet in spring, most bilious in summer and darkest in autumn.

8. In these circumstances it follows that the diseases which increase in winter should decrease in summer and *vice versa*. Those which come to an end in a given number of days are exceptions and I will discuss periodicity later on. You may expect diseases which begin in spring to end in the autumn; likewise autumnal diseases will disappear in the spring. Any disease which exceeds these limits must be put down as belonging to a whole year. In applying his remedies, the physician must bear in mind that each disease is most prominent during the season most in keeping with its nature.

9. In addition to these considerations, certain further points should be known. Diseases caused by over-eating are cured by fasting; those caused by starvation are cured by feeding up. Diseases caused by exertion are cured by rest; those caused by indolence are cured by exertion. To put it briefly; the physician should treat disease by the principle of opposition to the cause of the disease according to its form, its seasonal and age incidence, countering tenseness by relaxation and *vice versa*. This will bring the patient most relief and seems to me to be the principle of healing.

Some diseases are produced by the manner of life that is followed; others by the life-giving air we breathe. That there are these two types may be demonstrated in the following way. When a large number of people all catch the same disease at the same time, the cause must be ascribed to something common to all and which they all use; in other words to what they all breathe. In such a disease, it is obvious that individual bodily habits cannot be responsible because the malady attacks one after another, young and old, men and women alike, those who drink their wine neat and those who drink only water; those who eat barley-cake as well as those who live on bread, those who take a lot of exercise and those who take but little. The régime cannot therefore be responsible where people who live very different lives catch the same disease.

However, when many different diseases appear at the same time, it is plain that the regimen is responsible in individual cases. Treatment then should aim at opposing the cause of the disease as I have said elsewhere; that is, treatment should involve a change in regimen. For, in such a case, it is obvious that all, most, or at least one of the factors in the regimen does not agree with the patient; such must be sought out and changed having regard to the constitution of the patient, his age and appearance, the season of the year and the nature of the disease. The treatment prescribed should vary accordingly by lessening this or increasing that, and the regimen and drugs should be appropriately adapted to the various factors already mentioned.

When an epidemic of one particular disease is established, it is evident that it is not the regimen but the air breathed which is responsible. Plainly, the air must be harmful because of some morbid secretion which it contains. Your advice to patients at such a time should be not to alter the regimen since this is not to blame, but they should gradually reduce the quantity of food and drink taken so that the body is as little loaded and as weak as possible. A sudden change of regimen involves the risk of starting a fresh complaint, so you should deal with the regimen in this way when it is clearly not the cause of the patient's illness. Care should be taken that the amount of air breathed should be as small as possible and as unfamiliar as possible. These points may be dealt with by making the body thin so that the patient will avoid large and frequent breaths, and, wherever practicable, by a change of station from the infected area.

10. The most serious diseases are those which arise from the strongest part of the body, since if a disease remains in the place where it begins, it is inevitable that the whole body should sicken if its strongest part does. Alternatively, if the disease passes from the stronger part to a weaker part, it proves difficult to dispel. Those which pass from a weak part to a stronger are more easily cured because the in-flowing humours are easily spent by the strength of the part.

11. The blood-vessels of largest calibre, of which there are four pairs in the body, are arranged in the following way: one pair runs from the back of the head, through the neck and,

P

weaving its way externally along the spine, passes into the legs, traverses the calves and the outer aspect of the ankle, and reaches the feet. Venesection for pains in the back and loins should therefore be practised in the popliteal fossae or externally at the ankle.

The second pair of blood-vessels run from the head near the ears through the neck, where they are known as the jugular veins. Thence they continue deeply close to the spine on either side. They pass close to the muscles of the loins, entering the testicles and the thighs. Thence they traverse the popliteal fossa on the medial side and passing through the calves lie on the inner aspect of the ankles and the feet. Venesection for pain in the loin and in the testicles should therefore be done in the popliteal area or at the inner side of the ankle.

The third pair of blood-vessels run from the temples, through the neck and under the shoulder-blades. They then come together in the lungs; the right hand one crossing to the left, the left hand one crossing to the right. The right hand one proceeds from the lungs, passes under the breast and enters the spleen and the kidneys. The left hand one proceeds to the right on leaving the lungs, passes under the breast and enters the liver and the kidneys. Both vessels terminate in the anus.

The fourth pair run from the front of the head and the eyes, down the neck and under the clavicles. They then course on the upper surface of the arms as far as the elbows, through the forearms into the wrists and so into the fingers. They then return from the fingers running through the ball of the thumb and the forearms to the elbows where they course along the inferior surface of the arms to the axillae. Thence they pass superficially down the sides, one reaching the spleen and its fellow the liver. Thence they course over the belly and terminate in the pudendal area.

Apart from the larger vessels which are thus accounted for, there are a large number of vessels of all sizes running from the belly to all parts of the body; these carry foodstuffs to the body. They also form connections between the large main vessels which run to the belly and the rest of the body. In addition they anastomose with each other and form connections between the deep and superficial vessels.

The following are therefore rules for venesection. Care should be taken that the cuts are as close as possible to the determined source of the pain and the place where the blood collects. By doing this a sudden, violent change is avoided but at the same time the customary site of collection of blood will be changed.

12. If a patient over the age of thirty-five expectorates much without showing fever, passes urine exhibiting a large quantity of sediment painlessly, or suffers continuously from bloody stools, his complaint will arise from the following single cause. He must, when a young man, have been hard-working, fond of physical exertion and work and then, on dropping the exercises, have run to soft flesh very different from that which he had before. There must be a sharp distinction between his previous and his present bodily physique so that the two do not agree. If a person so constituted contracts some disease, he escapes for the time being but, after the illness, the body wastes. Fluid matter then flows through the blood-vessels wherever the widest way offers. If it makes its way to the lower bowel it is passed in the stools in much the same form as it was in the body; as its course is downward it does not stay long in the intestines. If it flows into the chest, suppuration results because, owing to the upward tread of its path, it spends a long time in the chest and there rots and forms pus. Should the fluid matter, however, be expelled into the bladder, it becomes warm and white owing to the warmth of that region. It becomes separated in the urine; the lighter elements float and form a scum on the surface while the heavier constituents fall to the bottom forming pus.

Children suffer from stones owing to the warmth of the whole body and of the vesical region in particular. Adult men do not suffer from stone because the body is cool; it should be thoroughly appreciated that a person is warmest the day he is born and coldest the day he dies. So long as the body is growing and advancing towards strength it is necessarily warm; but when it begins to wither and to fade away to feebleness, it cools down. From this principle it follows that a person is warmest the day he is born because he grows most on that day; he is coldest the day he dies because on that day he withers most.

People of the constitution mentioned above, that is athletic people who have got soft, generally recover of their own accord within forty-five days of the wasting beginning. If such a period be exceeded, natural recovery takes a year so long as no other malady intervenes.

13. Prognosis is safest to foretell in those diseases which develop quickly and those whose causes are apparent. They should be cured by opposing whatever is the cause of the disease, of which the body will thus be rid.

14. The presence of a sandy sediment or of stones in the urine means that originally tumours grew in relation to the aorta and suppurated. Then, because the tumour did not burst rapidly, stones were formed from the pus and these were squeezed out through the blood-vessels together with urine into the bladder. When the urine is only blood-stained, the blood-vessels have been attacked. Sometimes the urine is thick and small hair-like pieces of flesh are voided with it which, it must be realized, come from the kidneys and the joints. When, in an otherwise clear urine, a substance like bran is present in it, the bladder is inflamed.

15. Most fevers are caused by bile. Apart from those arising from local injury, they are of four types. These are called continued, quotidian, tertian and quartan.

Continued fever is produced by large quantities of the most concentrated bile and the crisis is reached in the shortest time; as the body enjoys no periods of coolness, the great heat it endures results in rapid wasting.

Quotidian fever is caused by a large quantity of bile, but less than that which causes continued fever. This is quicker than the others to depart although it lasts longer than a continued fever by as much as there is less bile causing it, and because the body has some respite from the fever whereas continued fever allows none.

Tertian fever lasts longer than quotidian fever and is caused by less bile. A tertian fever is longer in proportion to the longer respites from fever allowed to the body compared with quotidian fevers.

Quartans behave similarly to the tertians but last longer, as they arise from still less of the heat-producing bile and because they give the body longer respites in which to cool down. A secondary reason for their chronic character and difficult resolution is that they are caused by black bile; this is the most viscous of the humours in the body and remains the longest. As evidence of this note the association of quartan fevers with melancholy. Quartan fever has its highest incidence in the autumn and in those between the ages of twenty-five and forty-five. This is the time of life when the body is most subject to black bile, and the autumn is the corresponding season of the year. If a quartan fever occurs at any other time of the year, or at any other age, you may be sure that it will not be chronic unless some other malady be present.

A REGIMEN FOR HEALTH

An early recognition of the importance of preventive medicine.

1. The ordinary man should adopt the following regimen. During the winter, he should eat as much as possible, drink as little as possible and this drink should be wine as undiluted as possible. Of cereals, he should eat bread, all his meat and fish should be roasted and he should eat as few vegetables as possible during winter-time. Such a diet will keep the body warm and dry.

When spring comes, he should take more to drink, increasing the quantity and making it more watery, a little at a time. He should take softer cereals and less of them, substituting barley-cake for bread. Boiled meat should replace roast, and a few vegetables should be eaten once spring has begun. Thus will he effect a gradual change and towards the summer he will be taking a diet consisting entirely of soft cereals, boiled meat and vegetables both raw and boiled. At that time he will be taking the greatest quantity of the most diluted wine, taking care that the change is neither violent nor sudden but that it is made gradually.

During the summer he should live on soft barley-cake, watered wine in large quantities and take all his meat boiled. Such a diet is necessary in summer to make the body cool and soft, for the season, being hot and dry, renders the body burnt-up and parched, and such a condition may be avoided by a suitable diet. The change from spring to summer should follow the same pattern as that from winter to spring, decreasing the amount of cereals and increasing the quantity of drink taken.

A reversal of this process constitutes the transition from the summer to the winter diet. In the autumn the cereals should be increased and made drier, and likewise the meat in the diet. The quantity of drink taken should be decreased and taken less diluted so that he will have a good winter. Once more, then, he takes the smallest quantity of the least diluted drink and the largest quantity of cereals of the driest kind. This will keep him in good health and he will feel the cold less, for the season is cold and wet.

2. People with a fleshy, soft or ruddy appearance are best kept on a dry diet for the greater part of the year as they are constitutionally moist. Those with firm and tight-drawn skins, and those with tawny or dark complexions, should keep to a diet containing plenty of fluid most of the time, as the constitutions of such people are naturally dry. The softest and most moist diets suit young bodies best as at that age the body is dry and has set firm. Older people should take a drier diet most of the time, for at that age bodies are moist, soft and cold. Diets then must be conditioned by age, the time of year, habit, country and constitution. They should be opposite in character to the prevailing climate, whether winter or summer. Such is the best road to health.

3. In winter a man should walk quickly, in summer in more leisurely fashion unless he is walking in the hot sun. Fleshy people should walk faster, thin people more slowly. More baths should be taken in summer than in winter; firm people should bathe more than the fleshy ones. Garments in summer should be steeped in olive oil, but not in winter.

4. Fat people who want to reduce should take their exercise on an empty stomach and sit down to their food out of breath. They should not wait to recover their breath. They should before eating drink some diluted wine, not too cold, and their meat should be dished up with sesame seeds or seasoning and such-like things. The meat should also be fat as the smallest quantity of this is filling. They should take only one meal a day, go without baths, sleep on hard beds and walk about with as little clothing as maybe. Thin people who want to get fat should do exactly the opposite and never take exercise on an empty stomach.

5. The following rules are to be observed in the administration of emetics and enemata. Vomiting may be induced during the six winter months, as this is the phlegmatic time of year and diseases are centred about the head and in the chest.

During the warm weather, enemata may be used as this is the hot season when the body is more bilious and heaviness occurs in the loins and knees, when there are fevers and colic in the belly. It is necessary therefore to cool the body and draw downwards the matter surrounding those regions. For those who are rather fat and moist, use the thinner and more briny enemata; for those who are drier and have firmer flesh, use the more fatty and thicker enemata. By fatty and thicker enemas, I mean those made from milk and from chick-pea and boiled water and such-like; by thin and briny, such things as brine and sea-water.

Emetics should be administered as follows. Those who are fat, but not those who are lean, should vomit on an empty stomach after a run or a brisk walk about the middle of the day. The emetic should consist of a gill of ground hyssop in six pints of water; this should be drunk after adding vinegar and salt to improve the taste. It should at first be drunk slowly, but the remainder more quickly. Thinner and weaker people should take emetics after food in the following way. A hot bath should be followed by drinking half a pint of neat wine after which a meal of any kind of food should be taken, but no drink is taken either with the meal or after it. Wait as long as it takes to walk a mile and then administer a mixture of three wines, a bitter, a sweet and an acid one, at first neat in small doses at long intervals and then more diluted in larger doses and more frequently.

Those who are accustomed to induce vomiting twice a month will find it better to do so on two consecutive days rather than every fortnight; as it is, most people do the opposite. Those who benefit from vomiting and those who have difficulty with passing stools should eat several times a day and take all varieties of food and their meat cooked in every different way and drink two or three kinds of wine. The opposite kind of diet is best for those who do not indulge in vomiting or for those with relaxed bellies.

6. Infants should be bathed for long periods in warm water and given their wine diluted and not at all cold. The wine should be of a kind which is least likely to cause distension of

the stomach and wind. This should be done to prevent the occurrence of convulsions and to make the children grow and get good complexions. Women do best on a drier diet as dry foods are most suited to the softness of their flesh, and the less diluted drinks are better for the wombs and for pregnancy.

7. Those who enjoy gymnastics should run and wrestle during the winter; in summer, wrestling should be restricted and running forbidden, but long walks in the cool part of the day should take their place. Those who get exhausted with running should wrestle, and those who get exhausted with wrestling should run. By exercising in this way, the exhausted parts of the body will best be warmed, composed and rested.

Those who find that exercise causes diarrhoea and who pass undigested stools resembling food, should have their exercise cut by at least a third while their food should be halved. For it is clear that the belly cannot get sufficiently warm to digest the greater part of the food. The diet in such cases should consist of bread baked as well as possible together with wine that is practically undiluted. They should not walk after meals. They should also take only one meal a day during the time they have diarrhoea; this will give the belly the best chance to deal with the food that is given it. This sort of diarrhoea is most common in those who are particularly stout, when, their constitution being what it is, they are obliged to eat meat. The vessels being compressed, they cannot cope with the intake of food. This type of constitution is nicely balanced, liable to fall off in either direction and it is at its best for only a short time.

The sparer and more hirsute type of person can better cope with a big diet and also with hard exercise. They remain at the height of their powers for a longer period.

Those who vomit their food the day after it has been taken and suffer from distension of the hypochondrium showing that the food remains undigested, should take more sleep and force their bodies by exercise. They should drink more wine and take it less diluted and also, at these times, reduce the amount of food. For it is clear that the weakness and coldness of the belly prevent the greater part of the food from being digested.

Those who suffer from thirst should reduce both the amount of food and the amount of exercise they take, and they should be given watery wine to drink as cold as possible.

Those who get pains in the viscera as the result of gymnastics or any other form of exercise should rest without eating and drink the smallest quantity necessary to cause the passing of the greatest amount of urine. In this way the vessels coursing through the viscera will not become filled and distended and so cause tumours and fevers.

9.[1] A wise man ought to realize that health is his most valuable possession and learn how to treat his illnesses by his own judgement.

---

[1] Section 8, which is an interpolation from another work, is omitted.

COAN PROGNOSIS

This is an important collection of aphorisms derived from the Hippocratic school of medicine at Cos. Almost all its contents are repeated in another work entitled Prorrhetic, *but 'Coan Prognosis' has been selected for inclusion here as being the fuller of the two. It is probably slightly later than* Prorrhetic, *though still dating from the fifth century B.C. The compiler was clearly familiar with* Prognosis, *or more likely with a common source of the two works, for there are a number of parallel passages. This does not however detract from the importance of this collection, which now appears in English for the first time.*

(i)

1. Those in whom a rigor is followed by chilling, headache, pain in the neck, who lose their voice and sweat a little, although they may revive, will die.

2. It is when the sensation of illness is accompanied by severe chilling that it is of the worst significance.

3. Chilling combined with stiffening is fatal.

4. When fear and unexplained despondency follow chilling, a convulsion results.

5. When suppression of urine follows chilling, the significance is very bad.

6. It is bad when a rigor is followed by a state in which there is failure to recognize people; forgetfulness too is a bad sign.

7. Rigors accompanied by coma are somewhat dangerous, and flushing of the face with sweating is a bad sign in such cases. If chilling of the back supervenes on these symptoms, then a convulsion is provoked. It is a general rule, too, that convulsions are associated with chilling of the back.

8. Frequent attacks of shivering originating in the back and which pass rapidly to another part are bad; they denote the painful suppression of urine. A slight sweat in such cases is very bad.

9. A rigor taking place in the course of a continued fever, when the body is already weakened, is fatal.

10. Frequent slight sweating followed by rigors is fatal; terminally, both empyema and looseness of the bowels follow.

11. Rigors which originate in the back are the worst sort. Rigors which occur on the seventeenth day and recur on the twenty-fourth indicate difficult cases.

12. When the signs of shivering, headache and sweating are present together, it is bad.

13. Shivering with much sweating indicates a difficult case.

14. Frequent rigors associated with torpor are bad.

15. If a rigor occur on the sixth day, the crisis will be difficult.

16. Those who, in health, have frequent shivers develop an empyema after a haemorrhage.

17. Shivering and dyspnoea on exertion are signs of phthisis.

18. When, following empyema of the lung, occasional pains in the belly and about the clavicles are associated with râles and nausea, it denotes a large quantity of sputum in the lungs.

19. Those who suffer from shivering, nausea, lassitude and pain in the loins, are taken with a purging from the bowels.

20. Rigors, especially when the paroxysms occur towards nightfall, insomnia, babbling talk and, in some cases, incontinence of urine during sleep, end in a convulsion.

21. Continued rigors in acute disease are bad.

22. Headache and asthenia following upon a rigor is fatal; haematuria is also a bad sign in such cases.

23. A rigor accompanied by opisthotonus is fatal.

24. If a patient shiver and sweat as at a crisis, but then shivers next day contrary to expectation and also shows insomnia, then, the disease not having ripened, I expect a haemorrhage.

25. Suppression of urine accompanied by a rigor is bad and indicates a convulsion, especially if it be preceded by drowsiness. In such cases too, the parotids may be involved.

26. Rigors of tertian periodicity with paroxysms on alternate days, associated with irregular fever, are altogether bad.

27. A convulsion occurring with a rigor and fever is fatal.

28. Aphasia following a rigor is resolved by trembling; further rigors which are associated with trembling lead to a crisis.

29. Loss of strength with headache following a rigor denotes a dangerous condition. Haematuria is bad in such a case.

30. Rigors accompany suppression.

(ii)

31. During the course of a fever, convulsions and pain in the hands and feet are of bad significance; so also is a shooting pain from the thigh, while pain in the knees or in the calves is no better. In these cases there is sometimes delirium, especially if the urine contains suspended particles.

32. Fever following pain in the hypochondrium is bad; the worst thing is for drowsiness to supervene.

33. Failure of the fever to remit, with frequent slight sweating and a distended hypochondrium is, in most cases, bad. In such cases, pain located about the acromium and the clavicle is of serious significance.

34. It is bad when a tertian fever is associated with nausea.

35. Aphasia in fever is bad.

36. Lassitude, dim sight, insomnia, coma, a slight sweat, a rise in temperature—bad.

37. Lassitude with shivering, a slight sweat as at a crisis and then a return of warmth is bad in an acute disease, especially if there is epistaxis. About this time they show deep jaundice and die; in addition their stools are pale.

38. Erratic tertian fevers which change to the even days are difficult.

39. Tossing about with chilling but no sweating, on critical days, and all cases of restlessness unaccompanied by sweating and not at the crisis, are bad. It is also bad in a fever when rigors supervene with trembling and nausea and the vomiting of undigested bilious matter. It is also bad when the voice sounds as it does after a rigor.

40. Epistaxis accompanied by slight sweating and chilling is bad.

41. It is bad when slight sweating and sleeplessness is followed by a rise in temperature.

42. Slight sweating in a fever is a bad sign.

43. It is bad when the passage of bilious stools is associated with sharp pains about the chest and bitterness in the mouth.

44. In a fever it is bad if the belly be distended and unrelieved by the passage of wind.

45. Lassitude, hiccough, a fit—bad.

46. Slight sweating and with frequent slight shivering attacks starting in the back is bad, for it indicates a painful suppression of urine.

47. Doing something unusual, such as partaking of something unaccustomed, or not wanting to take something to which one is accustomed, is bad and not far removed from delirium.

48. Illnesses showing bad signs which improve, and those which show good signs yet do not, are difficult.

49. Slight sweating, especially about the head, together with malaise is bad in acute diseases, the more so if the urine be dark; in such cases too disturbed breathing is a bad sign.

50. Rapid alternation of heat and cold in the extremities, and similar alternations in thirst, are of bad significance.

51. A sharp retort from a polite person, in a high-pitched voice, is bad; in such cases, there is retraction of the hypochondrium.

52. A rapid increase in temperature following a cold sweat is of bad significance.

53. Slight sweating and a certain amount of discomfort are of bad significance in acute diseases.

54. Unexplained weakness in spite of sufficient nourishment is a bad sign.

55. In a fever, retching similar to that caused by vomiting, but which ends in clearing the throat and spitting is bad.

56. Rapid variations in sensation are bad.

57. Scanty epistaxes are bad.

58. It is in every way a bad sign if, in an acute disease, the desire to drink passes without drink being taken.

59. To jump on being touched, is bad.

60. When swellings come up in cases of *causus*-like fever, accompanied by drowsiness and stupor and pain down one side, the patient becomes paraplegic and dies.

61. Choking in acute cases associated with thinness is a fatal sign.

62. When the signs already suggest a fatal outcome, those who have slight trembling or rust-coloured vomit, those who take drink noisily and have rumblings if they take dry food, and those patients with dysphagia whose respiration is associated with cough, are in fatal case.

63. In acute diseases, redness of the hands and feet in a patient who is cold, is a fatal sign.

64. Those who puff and cry aloud in their sleep, half opening the eyes, die in deep jaundice, the stools becoming light-coloured.

65. When a febrile patient becomes demented and keeps silent although he has not lost the power to speak, it is fatal.

66. The appearance of livid patches in a fever denotes an early death.

67. Patients with fever who obtain relief following pain in the side by the passage of copious watery and bilious stools, but in whom this relief is followed by anorexia, bouts of sweating, a healthy look about the face, relaxed bowels and especially a pain in the heart; these, after a fairly long illness, die of pneumonia.

68. At the beginning of a fever the presence of black bile in the vomit or in the stools is a bad sign.

69. Those who are febrile yet chilled and who sweat slightly about the upper part of the body and experience discomfort, suffer from brain-fever and are in fatal case.

70. In an acute disease, brief stabs of pain about the clavicles and in the back are of fatal significance.

71. In long and fatal illness, a pain in the anus is a sign of death.

72. In those already in a weakened state, failure to hear, or distortion of the lip, eye or nostril, is a sign of death.

73. In fevers, pain in the groin indicates a long illness.

74. Failure of crises to develop in fevers prolongs the illness but is not fatal.

75. Fevers following on severe pains are long-lasting.

76. Dementia accompanied by trembling and groping denotes inflammation of the brain; . . .

77. When patients suffering from a continued fever lie speechless with their eyes closed but for an occasional flicker of the eyelids and then, after a nose bleed and vomiting, begin to speak and regain their wits, it is a sign they will recover. If these signs do not occur, they become dyspnoeic and soon die.

78. Fevers in which a paroxysm occurs on the second and fourth day of the disease, the third day being omitted, are bad. May it be that such paroxysms are due to disease of the brain?

79. When fevers depart on some day other than the critical ones, there is the chance of a relapse.

80. Those fevers which are slight at the start with throbbing of the head and thin urine, show an exacerbation towards the time of the crisis; it is not surprising to find that delirium and insomnia supervene as well.

81. In acute fevers, movements, tossing about or disturbed sleep may, in some cases, denote a convulsion.

82. Disturbed sleepless periods in which lack of restraint and wandering of the wits is shown are bad and denote a spasm, especially if associated with sweating. Chilling of the neck and back has similar associations, as also does chilling of the whole body and in these cases the urine contains membranous material.

83. Delirium with burning heat denotes a spasm.

84. Short unrestrained attacks of delirium are savage and also denote a spasm.

85. In long illnesses, unaccountable swellings in the belly denote a spasm.

86. Malaise at the start, insomnia and epistaxis; alleviation

at the sixth night but with pain next day; slight sweating, opening of the bowels, delirium—a copious haemorrhage and the end of the illness. Watery urine denotes an illness of this sort, if accompanied by the aforesaid signs.

87. To become distraught in melancholy fashion, and to begin to tremble, is bad.

88. Delirium with dyspnoea and sweating is a sign of death; so is dyspnoea and hiccough.

89. Dreams in cases of inflammation of the brain are distinctly seen.

90. In cases of inflammation of the brain, light-coloured stools and torpor are bad signs; a rigor is the worst sign of all.

91. In cases of inflammation of the brain, for the condition to be mild at the start, but to show frequent changes is bad.

92. It is a bad sign when a melancholic dementia is complicated by fits of trembling.

93. Are those who suffer from melancholic dementia and in whom trembling and expectoration supervenes, suffering from disease of the brain?

94. An acute fever supervening upon dementia, leads to inflammation of the brain.

95. Patients with disease of the brain drink little, are upset by noise and are liable to trembling fits and spasms.

96. Violent trembling in cases of disease of the brain is a sign of death.

97. Delirious behaviour in what relates to the necessities of life is the worst sort of delirium and, if this is followed by a paroxysm, the patient is in fatal case.

98. Wandering of the mind, a strident voice, spasm of the tongue and tremulousness indicates insanity. Stiffening is a fatal sign in these cases.

99. Delirium is more serious when the patient is already weakened.

100. Frequent changes in cases of inflammation of the brain, with spasms, are of bad significance.

101. Expectoration accompanied by chilling in cases of inflammation of the brain heralds the vomiting of dark material.

Q

102. In illnesses which have followed a varied course and which have involved wandering of the mind, frequently with coma, you may expect the vomiting of dark material.

103. Spasmodic paroxysms denote a seizure.

104. In protracted diseases, small dark haemorrhagic parotid swellings are of fatal significance.

105. Fevers associated with hiccough are fatal whether they be accompanied by ileus or not.

106. Large parotid swellings are seen in patients with dyspnoea who develop an acute fever with jaundice and a distended hypochondrium, after being chilled.

107. When, in cases of fever, pain in the loins and in the lower parts of the body spreads to the region of the diaphragm, it is a fatal sign especially if some other bad sign appears as well; if the other signs, however, are not bad, there is a chance that an empyema may be formed.

108. In infants suffering from acute fevers; constipation and insomnia, kicking out with the legs, change of colour and flushing red, herald a fit.

109. Restlessness at the onset of an illness with insomnia and the passage of dark solid stools sometimes indicate haemorrhage.

110. Insomnia with sudden restlessness indicates haemorrhage, especially if there has previously been blood loss. May this not also happen after a chill?

111. To be chilled for a short while and to sweat a little, and to cough about the times of paroxysms of the disease is of bad significance; if pain in the side and a sense of suffocation supervene, it means that an empyema has formed.

112. The appearance of a generalized pustular rash in cases of continued fever is a sign of death unless some localizing abscess be formed; such an abscess commonly appears near the ear.

113. In acute fevers it is bad to be chilled externally but to burn inside and to be thirsty.

114. Continued fevers becoming more acute every third day are dangerous; but once the fever remits, there is no further danger.

115. In protracted fevers, swelling or pain in the joints may occur; they are not without profit.

116. In acute fevers, the onset of headache and distension of the hypochondrium may lead to brain-fever, unless there is an epistaxis.

117. Malignant intermittent fevers do not resolve unless cholera supervenes.

118. Jaundice occurring before the seventh day of the disease is bad, but when it appears on the seventh, ninth, eleventh and fourteenth it denotes the crisis, so long as it does not produce a hardening of the hypochondrium; occurring otherwise, its meaning is ambiguous.

119. Frequent relapses with a repetition of the same signs with vomiting about the time of the crisis, result in the vomiting of dark material and trembling.

120. When paroxysms of pain occur simultaneously with the exacerbation of fever in tertian fevers, they result in the passage of clots of blood in the stools.

121. In fevers, pulsation and pain in the blood vessels of the neck, ends in dysentery.

122. Frequent changes of colour and temperature are useful.

123. Acute bilious fevers, heavy breathing and distension of the hypochondrium, result in swelling of the parotids.

124. Convalescents who eat well but fail to put on weight have a bad relapse.

125. Temporal pulsation, a healthy complexion and lack of suppleness of the hypochondrium in cases of fever, indicate a prolonged illness. Such fevers do not resolve unless there be a copious epistaxis, hiccough, a convulsion, or pain in the hips.

126. In *causus*, violent diarrhoea is a sign of death.

127. The onset of fever like that of *causus* following violent pain in the belly, is a fatal sign.

128. In fevers of the *causus* type, ringing noises in the head associated with dimness of vision and a heavy feeling in the nose indicate the onset of melancholic dementia unless epistaxis occurs.

129. In cases of *causus*, trembling is ended by the onset of delirium.

130. In cases of *causus*, an epistaxis taking place on the fourth day is a bad sign unless it be accompanied by some other sign which is favourable; occurring on the fifth day it is less dangerous.

131. Cases of *causus* type associated with slight chilling, frequent watery and bilious stools and difficulty of vision are bad ones, especially if a seizure occurs.

132. *Causus* is resolved by a rigor.

133. Cases of *causus* are usually recurrent; after exhibiting the symptoms for four days a sweat follows, if not, this occurs on the seventh day.

134. Fourteen days mark the crisis in fever of the *causus* type, bringing either alleviation or death.

135. No cases of *causus* recover unless an abscess appears in the parotid region.

136. Patients who suffer from drowsiness, showing twitching of the hands and sleepiness, are of bad colour and liable to oedema, while the pulse is sluggish and the parts under the eyes swollen. They also have attacks of sweating and they are incontinent of their stools which are bilious or very dry. Urine and stools are passed copiously, the former resembling that of cattle. They ask neither food nor drink. When they regain consciousness, they complain of pain in the neck and noises in the ears. Those who recover from this condition of drowsiness usually have an empyema.

(iii)

137. In fevers where shivering stops at other times than at a crisis, later on an aching abscess appears at one of the joints, and the bladder is painful.

138. Febrile patients with a flushed face, severe headache and pulsating blood vessels, usually have a haemorrhage; those who have nausea, heartburn and expectoration, usually have vomiting. Those who have belching, wind, borborygmi and swellings usually have some upset of the bowels.

139. In those cases where a continued fever lasts a long time without danger in the absence of pain or inflammation, or any other obvious cause, expect the formation of an abscess

accompanied by pain and swelling especially in the lower parts of the body. Such an abscess should particularly be expected in patients up to thirty years old; in such persons suspect an abscess if the fever lasts more than twenty days. They occur less often with older people, even if the fever lasts a long time. Fevers which intermit and recur irregularly are especially likely to change to a quartan when autumn comes, more particularly in those over thirty. In winter, abscess formation occurs more often, stops more slowly and is less liable to recur.

140. If frequent recurrences of fever go on for more than six months, wasting about the hips is likely to occur.

141. All signs of change in the course of a fever, which do not indicate the localization of an abscess, are bad.

142. Fevers which depart neither on the critical days, nor with the signs of resolution, recur.

143. Acute diseases reach a crisis in fourteen days.

144. An exact tertian reaches a crisis in five, or in seven, or at most, in nine periods.

145. If at the beginning of a fever there is an epistaxis, or sneezing, and the urine contains a white sediment on the fourth day, this indicates resolution on the seventh day.

146. Acute diseases reach a crisis: if an epistaxis occur on a critical day and much sweating takes place, if purulent urine is passed or plenty of clear urine with a favourable sediment, if an abscess of considerable size appear, if the stools contain blood and mucus and are passed precipitately, and if there is vomiting without distress about the expected time of the crisis.

147. Undisturbed deep sleep denotes a safe crisis; disturbed sleep with bodily pain, an unsure one.

148. Epistaxis taking place on the seventh, ninth or fourteenth days usually ends a fever; the same is true of bilious and dysenteric conditions of the bowels, pain in the knees or hips, and in the passing of ripe urine towards the crisis, and, in the case of women, the onset of menstruation.

149. Those who, during the course of a fever, suffer from bleeding from any part of the body whatsoever, have relaxed bowels during their convalescence.

150. Patients with fevers who suffer from slight sweating, headache and constipation are liable to spasms.

151. Brief bold bouts of delirium denote a fierce disease and a fit.

152. A spasm occurring in a fever stops it the same day, or the next day, or the day after.

153. A spasm occurring during the course of a fever and ceasing the same day is good; but if it lasts longer than an hour without intermission, it is bad.

154. Those who suffer from irregularly intermittent fevers, the belly being distended and the stools scanty, develop pain in the loins and acute diarrhoea about the time of the crisis. Those whose hands are burning hot, who are sluggish, thirsty, nauseated and constipated and who feel oppressed, turn yellow. Sometimes a bright red inflammation of the feet has the same significance.

155. Winter quartan fevers are pretty likely to change to acute diseases.

(iv)

156. Intense headache associated with another unfavourable sign in cases of acute fever is a sign of death. If there be no other unfavourable sign and it lasts more than twenty days, it denotes epistaxis or discharge of pus from the nose, or of abscess formation in the lower parts of the body. You should expect discharges of blood or pus more especially in people under thirty-five; abscess formation in the case of older people, but discharges if the pain is around the face and temples.

157. When patients who are not febrile complain of headache and noises in the head, vertigo, slowness of speech and numbness of the hands, expect them to become either epileptic or to suffer from apoplexy, or to suffer from loss of memory.

158. Patients with headache who show delirium and fits, constipation, staring eyes and a suffused complexion develop opisthotonus.

159. Head-shaking, intense redness of the eyes and being plainly delirious, are fatal signs; such signs do not continue till death, but result in parotid swellings.

160. Headache accompanied by pain in the perineum and genitalia results in torpor and incontinence of urine and enfeebles the voice. These symptoms are not troublesome but the patient then becomes drowsy and liable to hiccough. In the ninth month after the onset, the voice being regained, the symptoms reappear owing to the patient being infected with ascaris.

161. Headache followed by deafness and coma results in a swelling in the neighbourhood of the ear.

162. Those who suffer from headache and distress as in a seizure with very red eyes, are liable to haemorrhage.

163. Shaking the head and the presence of noises in the head indicates a haemorrhage or, in the case of women, menstrual discharge, especially if a hot feeling along the spine follows—perhaps also dysentery.

164. Those with heaviness of the head and pain in the frontal region and insomnia, are liable to haemorrhage, especially if there is also some tension in the neck.

165. In cases of headache, the vomiting of rust-coloured matter accompanied by deafness and insomnia, quickly leads to madness.

166. Cases of pain in the head and neck, and a certain weakness and twitching of the whole body, are ended by a haemorrhage. However, they may also resolve in the course of time although meanwhile there is retention of urine.

167. Acute headaches and those accompanied by numbness and a feeling of heaviness, are frequently followed by spasms.

168. Headache is resolved by the discharge of pus from the nose, by the production of thick odourless sputum, by the eruption of sores, and sometimes by sleep or by the passage of a diarrhoeic stool.

169. Moderate headache accompanied by thirst, but without sweating or with sweating that does not terminate the fever, denotes gingival abscesses, or abscess near the ear, so long as there is no bowel upset.

170. A headache accompanied by drowsiness and heaviness brings on a liability to spasms.

171. Are those with headache, thirst, slight insomnia,

dysphasia, weakness and lassitude following relaxed bowels, liable to dementia?

172. Those with headache, slight deafness, shaking of the hands, pain in the neck, dark and cloudy urine, and dark vomit, are in fatal case.

173. Those with headache, slight sweating and constipation are liable to spasms.

174. Drowsiness is altogether bad.

175. Are those who become comatose at the beginning of an illness, with pain in the head, loins, neck, hypochondrium, and insomnia, suffering from disease of the brain? Drops of blood from the nostrils in such cases is a fatal sign, especially if this occur on the fourth day or at the start. A very red discharge from the bowels is also bad.

176. Those are in fatal case who from the start have slight sweats, 'ripe' urine, feverishness but cool off at times other than the critical ones, and who at frequent intervals become very hot, torpid and comatose and liable to spasms.

177. Coma-like sleep and acute chilling are fatal signs.

178. Those who suffer from coma, lassitude, deafness and acute diarrhoea, are helped by the passage of red stools around the time of the crisis.

179. Those who suffer from coma, nausea, pain in the hypochondrium and the vomiting of small quantities, suffer from swellings near the ears but, earlier, swelling of the face.

180. Conditions accompanied by coma, with sudden delirium and flinging the limbs about, are likely to result in haemorrhage.

181. States of coma associated with nausea, pain in the hypochondrium and the frequent expectoration of a small amount of sputum, lead to parotid swellings. Is there some connection between coma and spasms?

182. In cases of coma, dementia, fits, variations in the condition of the hypochondrium and abdominal tumours, anorexia, constipation and slight sweating, does disturbed respiration and the passage of something resembling semen denote the onset of hiccough? And does the passage of

bilious stools follow? The passage of urine with a scum on it is advantageous; in these cases the bowels are upset.

(v)

183. Following mortification of the brain, some die in three days, some in seven; if seven days are survived, then recovery follows. Those cases die in which, on making an incision, loss of bone is discovered.

184. A copious thick epistaxis is bad for those with headache associated with fracture of the bones of the back of the skull; these patients have rigors preceded by a pain in the eyes. Are fractures of the temporal bones liable to produce spasms?

(vi)

185. Intense ear-ache with acute fever and one of the other bad signs, proves fatal to young people in seven days or fewer, unless there is a copious discharge of pus from the ear, or epistaxis, or some other favourable sign. Death is preceded by delirium. In the case of older people, the illness is less acute and less fatal as there is longer in which the ear may discharge pus. Also, old people are less liable to delirium; nevertheless most of them relapse and then die.

186. The onset of deafness in the course of acute difficult illnesses is a bad sign; it is also bad in protracted cases for in these it also brings on pains in the hips.

187. In fevers, deafness checks diarrhoea.

188. It is a fatal sign if the ears be cold, translucent and contracted.

189. Buzzing and noises in the ears is a sign of death in acute diseases.

190. Noises in the head with dimness of vision and a heavy feeling in the nose is a sign of delirium, and leads to haemorrhage.

191. Those who suffer from deafness with heaviness of the head, distension of the hypochondrium and photophobia, have a haemorrhage.

192. In an acute fever, the onset of deafness indicates dementia.

193. To be hard of hearing, to show tremor in picking up anything, to have a paralysed tongue, to be sluggish—is bad.

194. It is a sign of delirium when, following a period of ill health, deafness supervenes and the urine is reddish with particles suspended in it but fails to form a sediment. Jaundice is bad in such cases, as is imbecility supervening on the jaundice. It sometimes happens that the patient loses the power of speech without losing consciousness; the belly may also be in a bad state.

195. Swellings near the ear accompanied by pain constitute a fatal sign.

196. In a fever, aching near the ear followed by the appearance of red patches is a sign of an oncoming attack of erysipelas of the face. But spasms accompanied by loss of voice and feebleness also follow these signs.

197. Parotid swelling supervening upon evil-smelling ileus, acute fever and prolonged distension of the hypochondrium, are fatal.

198. Swelling by the ear is bad for the paralytic.

199. Swellings by the ear in protracted illnesses are a sign of death unless they discharge pus; the bowels are relaxed in such cases.

200. In patients with swellings by the ear, do they have headache? Do they have slight sweats about the upper parts of the body? Do they also have rigors following these things? Do they have violent diarrhoea? And are they comatose at all? Is the urine watery with white matter suspended in it? And are the stools somewhat varied, being very pale in colour and foul-smelling?

201. Swellings by the ear are made to discharge by a slight cough accompanied by expectoration.

202. In cases of swelling by the ears, it is a bad sign when the urine quickly becomes 'ripe' and stays so only for a short while; to have a fit of chilling in these circumstances is very bad.

203. In protracted illness, swellings by the ear are fatal which, although they suppurate, produce pus which is not

very white in colour and which is odourless, especially in women.

204. Parotid swellings occur most often in acute illnesses of the *causus* group. Unless they ripen and precipitate a crisis, or there is an epistaxis, or the urine shows a thick deposit, the patients die. The majority of such swellings clear up. In addition, you should keep an eye on the fever, whether it increases or remits, and propound an opinion accordingly.

205. A dripping from the nose supervening upon deafness or torpor indicates some difficulty; in such cases vomiting and purging is useful.

206. Swellings by the ears are very likely to follow on deafness, especially if there by any sensation of nausea; they are even more likely to arise if the patients are comatose as well.

207. Deafness occurring in a fever is ended by an epistaxis or a disturbance of the bowels.

(vii)

208. When the face, from being swollen, becomes thin again, when the voice becomes softer and quieter, when the respirations become less frequent and shallower—it is a sign of a remission the following day.

209. Falling-in of the face is a sign of death; though less so if caused by insomnia, fasting or diarrhoea. If these be the cause of the falling-in, it recovers in twenty-four hours. The signs are: the eyes hollow, the nose sharp, the temples fallen in, the ears cold and contracted, the skin hard, the colour pale or dark. If, in addition to these signs, the eyelid, lip or nose become livid, death is at hand.

210. A good colour to the face and scowling in an acute disease is bad; when contraction of the forehead follows on these signs, it denotes brain-fever.

211. A good colour and sweating about the face in the absence of fever, indicates a failure to excrete old waste products, or irregularity of régime.

212. Redness of the nose is a sign of looseness of the bowels.

212a. Pain or suppuration in the hypochondrium or in the lungs is of bad significance.

(viii)

213. It is a sign of the crisis when the eyes and their whites, having been dark or livid, become clear. To become clear quickly denotes a quick crisis; slowly, a tardy one.

214. For the eyes to become misty, or for the whites to become red or livid or to show marked venous congestion, is not a pretty sign; it is also a poor sign when there is photophobia, or lachrymation, or strabismus, or if one pupil becomes smaller than the other. It is also bad if the eyes move restlessly, or if there are small styes, or if they show a thin skin over them, or if the pupil becomes smaller and the white of the eye bigger, or if the pupil is hidden by the upper eyelid. Bad signs too are enophthalmos, a severe degree of exophthalmos, lack of their lustre so that the pupil fails to dilate, irregularity of the eyelids, fixity of the eyes, continuous blinking and changes of colour. For the eyes not to close in sleep is a fatal sign. Squint is also bad.

215. Redness of the eyes occurring during the course of a fever denotes protracted stomach trouble.

216. Swellings by the eyes in convalescence indicate violent diarrhoea.

217. A rigor supervening on strabismus of the eyes, with lassitude and fever, is a fatal sign. To be comatose when these signs are present is bad also.

218. Fever supervening on ophthalmia ends the latter; if it does not, there is risk of losing one's sight, or one's life, or both.

219. When headache develops in cases of ophthalmia and accompanies it for a long time, there is a risk of blindness.

220. Spontaneous diarrhoea in ophthalmia is advantageous.

221. Dimness of vision with fixity and mistiness of the eyes, is bad.

222. Dimness of vision associated with loss of consciousness, indicates that a convulsion will shortly follow.

223. Fixity of the eyes in an acute fever, or sharp movements

with disturbed sleep or insomnia, and sometimes associated with slight epistaxis, have nothing good about them. If the subject is not burning hot to the touch, he succumbs to brain-fever, especially if there is haemorrhage.

(ix)

224. The tongue being tremulous at first, but retaining its colour, then later becoming rough, livid and fissured, is a sign of death; if it becomes very dark, it indicates that the crisis will take place on the fourteenth day. It is of worst significance when it is either black or yellow.

225. If the tongue have the appearance of being smeared along the median raphe with white grease, it is a sign of remission in a fever. If the matter formed on it be thick, the remission will occur the same day; if thinner, the next; if still thinner, the day after. It has the same significance if the fur appears at the tip of the tongue but less so.

226. Tremulousness of the tongue together with redness about the nose and relaxed bowels, in the absence of any abnormal signs in the lungs, is of bad significance and indicates fatal diarrhoea.

227. Abnormal softness of the tongue, together with nausea and cold sweats following relaxation of the bowels, is a sign of the vomiting of dark material. Lassitude is bad in such cases.

228. Tremulous tongues are, in some patients, associated with relaxed bowels; if the tongue turns black, it indicates speedy death. Is a tremulous tongue a sign that the wits are wandering?

229. A shaggy, very dry tongue is a sign of brain-fever.

(x)

230. To gnash or grind the teeth, unless this has been a habit from childhood, is a sign of madness and death. If a patient who is already out of his mind does this, then it is certainly fatal. It is also fatal when the teeth become dry.

231. Mortification of a tooth brings an end to a gingival abscess.

232. When severe fever and delirium supervene on mortification of a tooth, it is a sign of death. If recovery takes place, there will be suppurating ulcers and sequestration of the bone.

233. When the palate becomes oedematous, it usually suppurates.

234. There is the danger, when there is violent pain in the jaws, that there will be sequestrum formation in the bone.

235. Pursing of the lip denotes a bilious flux of the bowels.

236. Bleeding from the gums on top of relaxed bowels is a fatal sign.

(xi)

237. In a fever, the hawking up of sputum which is livid, dark and bilious, is bad if the sputum be retained; if the sputum comes away normally, it is a useful happening.

238. Those who have a cough with salty sputum, show a pustular efflorescence of the complexion which, before death, becomes roughened.

239. Frequent hawking, if accompanied by any of the other signs, denotes brain-fever.

(xii)

240. Aphonia is of the most serious significance if accompanied by weakness.

241. Short bold fits of delirium are bad and denote a fierce disease.

242. Those who develop aphonia while febrile but not at a critical time, die with tremor.

243. Aphonia during a fever in the manner of that seen in a seizure, associated with a quiet delirium, is fatal.

244. Pain, then aphonia—a hard death.

245. Aphonia with a seizure is fatal.

246. A cracked voice after purging—is this bad? Most patients in this case have slight sweating and their bellies become relaxed.

247. In cases of aphonia, the presence of that type of breathing seen in suffocation is bad—is it also a sign of delirium?

248. Aphonia, following headache accompanied by sweating, fever, incontinence of the stools, and then remitting, denotes a prolonged illness. A rigor supervening in such cases is not a bad sign.

249. Cases of dementia accompanied by aphonia prove fatal.

250. Aphonia in patients who have rigors is a sign of death; they usually suffer from headache.

251. Aphonia accompanied by weakness in an acute fever is a sign of death in the absence of sweating, but is of less serious significance if sweating be present, when it denotes a long illness. It may be that these signs are safest when they are seen during a relapse; those are most likely to die who have epistaxis and those who have diarrhoea.

252. A shrill whining voice and dimness of the eyes denote a spasm; pains in the lower parts of the body in such cases show that they will get over it.

253. Unexpected diarrhoea accompanied by a quavering voice is a fatal sign in complaints which have lasted a long time.

254. Frequent attacks of aphonia with slight stupor foretells a consumptive condition.

(xiii)

255. Rapid shallow respiration denotes inflammation and pain in the vital parts; slow deep respiration indicates delirium or a seizure. Cold breath is a sign of death; so also is feverish and smoky breath, but less so than cold. Prolonged expiration and a small inspiration, short expiration and prolonged inspiration, are the worst kinds and nearest to death. Prolonged, hurried faint and bi-phasic inspiration (as if they were breathing in again) are of similar significance. The presence of eupnoea carries considerable weight as a factor denoting recovery from all conditions seen in acute fevers, even if it takes forty days to reach a crisis.

(xiv)

256. The neck hard and painful, the laws locked together, a violent throbbing of the jugular veins, and contraction of the muscles, is fatal.

257. Choking pains in a neck not affected by swelling and starting from a headache, indicate a spasm.

258. Chilling of the neck and back, which seems to spread over the whole body, denotes a spasm; in these cases the urine contains particles like barley-meal.

259. Those with irritation of the pharynx generally have swellings near the ears.

260. A pharynx which is not swollen but which is painful and distressing is highly fatal.

261. Those whose breath is drawn in, whose voice is as if choked, and whose axis vertebra is sunk in, these cases have breathing as the end approaches like one who is convulsive.

262. The throat slightly roughened, ineffective motions of the bowels, frontal headache, carphology, pain: an increase in any of these symptoms indicates a difficult illness.

263. Violent pain in the throat produces swellings near the ears and spasms.

264. Pains in both the neck and back accompanied by acute fever and a spasm, are fatal.

265. Pain in the neck and forearms indicates a spasm; it originates in the face and around the neck. Patients in this condition are usually pale and thin and expectorating, and it is good for them to sweat while sleeping—may it be that to be helped by a sweat is not bad for most people? Pains in the lower part of the body are easily borne by these patients.

266. In cases of pain in the back and chest, the passing of bloody urine turning into anuria indicates a distressing illness ending fatally.

267. Pain in the neck, always of bad significance in all fevers, is worst where there is a chance of the patient going mad.

268. Disturbed bowels associated with torpor, supervening on pain in the chest with fever, is a sign of melaena.

269. Where a patient suffering from an acute illness develops a slightly painful condition of the throat in which he has difficulty in closing the mouth after opening it, and where there is no swelling, it denotes delirium. If he develops brain-fever after showing these signs, it is fatal.

270. Ulceration of the throat with fever, attended by any of the other signs of bad significance, is dangerous.

271. In fevers, in the absence of swelling, it is bad to choke suddenly and to be unable to swallow.

272. To be unable to turn the neck or to swallow is generally a sign of death.

(xv)

273. The hypochondrium should be soft, painless and smooth. If it is inflamed, or uneven, or painful, it is a sign of no slight illness.

274. A swelling which is hard and painful in the hypochondrium is of very bad significance if it extend over the whole area; but if it is on one side only, a swelling on the left is less dangerous. At the beginning of an illness such a swelling denotes an early death, but if the patient lasts more than twenty days, the fever being maintained, the formation of an empyema occurs. These patients may suffer from epistaxis during the first period, and this is very beneficial for they generally have pains in the head and dulled vision. Epistaxis is especially to be expected to occur in such cases, at least with those under thirty-five years of age, though it is less likely with older patients.

275. The presence of soft and painless swellings cause the crisis to be retarded but are less dangerous. These too, if they last more than sixty days while the fever is maintained, indicate the formation of an empyema. Swellings about the belly have much the same significance as those in the hypochondrium, except that they are less likely to indicate empyema; least of all, those below the navel. These empyemata are encapsulated, but some are diffuse. Any that rupture internally prove fatal. Of the remaining empyemata, those that rupture externally are best if they become sharply and strictly localized. Those that are internal are best if they produce no swelling, pain or discoloration. The opposite is the worst. Some of these give no indication of their presence on account of the thickness of the pus. Swellings of recent origin in the hypochondrium, unless accompanied by inflammation, are ended, together

R

with the pain they produce, if rumbling occurs in the hypo-chondrium, especially if this should be evacuated through the urine and stools, or, alternatively, is discharged by itself; it is also beneficial if this descends to the lower parts of the body.

276. Throbbing in the hypochondrium with distress heralds delirium, especially if there are frequent movements of the eye.

277. Pain in the heart and throbbing in the hypochondrium, the fever having given way to chilling, is bad especially if there is slight sweating.

278. Pains seizing on the hypochondrium are specially bad if they produce relaxation of the bowels; and they are worse if the onset be acute. Parotid swelling following is a bad sign, as are other examples of suppuration.

279. Cardalgia with colic indicates the expulsion of intestinal worms.

280. Frequent attacks of pain in the heart in an old person often denote sudden death.

281. Distension of the hypochondrium, the bowels being constipated, is bad; this is specially true in consumptive patients, who have been ill a long time and in those whose bowels were previously relaxed.

282. A suppurating area of inflammation in the hypochon-drium causes, in some cases, the passage of dark stools before death.

283. Distension of the hypochondrium associated with nausea, coma and headache, leads to parotid swellings.

284. In bilious patients, the onset of heavy breathing and acute fever following swelling in the hypochondrium, causes parotid swellings.

285. In febrile cases where there is pain in the hypochon-drium with slight rumbling, the onset of pain in the loins generally relaxes the bowels, unless flatus or a large quantity of urine is passed.

286. Parotid abscess supervening on chronic swelling of the hypochondrium with fetid stools is fatal.

287. In cases of pain in the hypochondrium, the passage, little by little, of small viscous dung-like stools indicates jaundice. Do they also indicate a haemorrhage?

288. Sudden pain in the region of the hypochondrium and heart, unattended by fever, and extending into the lower part of the body and the legs, is ended by venesection or purging. It is harmful when such patients become feverish, as the fevers become chronic and violent, and cough, heavy breathing and hiccough occur. When these are about to terminate, there may be violent pain in the hips or legs, or an expectoration of pus, or loss of vision may supervene.

289. When a patient suffers from pain in the hypochondrium, heart, liver and the parts round the umbilicus, he will recover if he passes blood in the stools, but if not, he will die.

290. Illnesses attended with a vigorous complexion of the face and not showing softness of the hypochondrium, do not terminate without copious epistaxis or a spasm or pain in the hips.

291. Pain in the region of the hypochondrium in fevers where the patients have lost their voices, when the pain resolves without sweating, are bad. In such cases, the pains go to the hips.

292. Throbbing in the belly in cases of fever brings on delirium, while a haemorrhage produces shivering.

293. Violent diarrhoea taking place during the course of a fever of *causus* type is fatal.

294. Throbbing pains in the region of the navel have some connection with delirium, but about the time of the crisis in such cases, thick mucus is passed in the stools, often with pain.

296.[1] Those patients with an affection of the hypochondrium who show tossing about, die consequent upon the appearance of parotid swellings.

297. Pain in the belly associated with rigidity, and accompanied by fever, shivering, anorexia and some relaxation of the bowels not amounting to a purging, end in the formation of empyemata.

(xvi)

298. Pain in the epigastrium and an ache in the loins which are not resolved by the administration of a purge, end in a dry dropsy.

[1] No. 295 is omitted as being merely a repetition of No. 281.

299. Aching pains in the loins of long duration associated with paroxysms of fever of tertian periodicity, result in the passage in the stools of clots of blood.

300. Pain in the loin indicates haemorrhage from the bowels.

301. Haemorrhage from the bowels following pain in the loins is copious.

302. Where pain in the loins is followed by pain in the head, numbness of the hands, cardalgia and noises in the ears, there is a violent haemorrhage from the bowels, severe diarrhoea and, generally, some mental disturbance.

303. Illnesses starting with pain in the back run a difficult course.

304. In cases of intense pain in the back, more than the patient can bear, the vomiting of a lot of frothy material as the result of taking hellebore, is beneficial.

305. Deformity of the spine with dyspnoea is resolved by a haemorrhage.

306. When cardalgia supervenes on, or precedes, a case of pain in the loins, it is a sign of haemorrhage from the bowels.

307. Pains passing from the loins to the head and neck and associated with a sort of paralysis, indicate spasms and delirium. Do spasms end these pains? Or are the bellies of those who suffer these things diseased?

308. Pains ascending from the loins and associated with squinting of the eyes is bad.

309. It is bad when a patient suffering from pain in the chest shows torpor; supervening on a fever, it means a rapid death.

310. Pain ascending from the loins to the heart accompanied by fever, shivering and the vomiting up of a small amount of thin watery material, indicates that the patient will die following delirium marked by aphonia and the vomiting of dark material.

311. Long-standing aching in the loins, in the small intestine, and pain in the region of the hypochondrium, along with anorexia and fever, mean that if an intense ache comes to the head, death will occur acutely in the manner of a spasm.

312. Those with pains in the loins are in a bad way; do they suffer from trembling and is their voice as in a rigor?

313. Is there a chance that those with lumbar pain, nausea, no vomiting and a few fits of severe delirium, may pass dark stools?

314. Pain in the loins with cardalgia and violent expectoration has some suggestion of a spasm.

315. Dysphasia may occur with a rigor at the time of crisis.

316. Frequently recurrent pain in the loins without obvious cause is a sign of serious illness.

317. Lumbar pain associated with burning heat and nausea is bad.

318. Tension in the loins following a copious menstrual discharge, is a sign of abscess formation. Of similar significance is the onset of various kinds of discharge, mucoid or foul-smelling, when accompanied by choking, following on copious menstruation as mentioned before. I think that such women also have slight delirium.

319. Those who have pain in the loins and flank without obvious reason become jaundiced.

(xvii)

320. Intense chilling following haemorrhage on a critical day is the very worst kind.

321. Contralateral haemorrhage is bad; e.g. epistaxis from the right nostril in the case of an enlarged spleen, and similarly with other swellings in the hypochondrium.

322. Haemorrhagic wounds followed by rigors are of serious significance and patients suffering from them die unexpectedly while talking.

323. Copious haemorrhage on the fifth day of the disease, with rigors occurring on the sixth and chilling on the seventh, and this followed by a sharp rise of temperature, means that they have stomach trouble.

324. The passage of dark stools following haemorrhage is of bad significance; so also are very red stools. Such haemorrhages take place on the fourth day, the patients becoming first

comatose and then having spasms before they die; previously they have passed dark stools and show abdominal distension.

325. Deafness associated with haemorrhage and melaena during the course of an acute illness is of bad significance; the passage of blood is a fatal sign, but it ends the deafness.

326. Those who have recurrent haemorrhages suffer from stomach trouble as time goes on unless 'ripe' urine be passed. Does watery urine also have some such significance?

327. In those cases where large dark stools are passed following frequent and copious haemorrhage, and when these have stopped there is haemorrhage from the bowels, the patients suffer pain in the belly which is relieved by the emission of wind. Do such patients have frequent but mild bouts of sweating with many cold fits? Disturbed urine is not a bad sign in these cases; nor is it when it shows a scum like semen, but generally those people pass watery urine.

328. Cases where slight epistaxis follows deafness and torpor are somewhat difficult in their course; vomiting and an upset of the bowels help.

329. Large haemorrhages at the beginning of an illness cause relaxed bowels in convalescence.

330. It sometimes provokes a spasm when a copious epistaxis is stopped by force; venesection puts an end to it.

331. When epistaxis occurs on the eleventh day, it is a sign of a difficult illness; especially if it happens twice.

332. Either hiccough or a spasm following a large flow of blood is a bad sign.

333. When children of seven years of age show weakness, a bad colour and rapid respiration on walking, together with a desire to eat earth, it denotes destruction of the blood and asthenia.

334. In long illnesses the occurrence of small haemorrhages from the bowels is a fatal sign.

335. Vertigo at the start of an illness is ended by epistaxis.

336. Epistaxis accompanied by small sweats with chilling is of bad significance.

337. Venesection of a torpid chilled patient is bad.

338. When haemorrhage attends constipation, and rigors

attend the haemorrhage, the patients' bellies become disturbed and somewhat hard, or the patient is suffering from ascaris, or both conditions may occur together.

339. When haemorrhages from the bowel occur at regular intervals accompanied by thirst, cessation of the haemorrhages brings about death from fits.

340. Dizziness immediately following a haemorrhage from the bowels denotes a slight and temporary paralysis which may be ended by venesection. Nevertheless, such a happening must be regarded as a bad sign.

(xviii)

341. Do those who palpitate all over die with aphonia?

342. Trembling turning into a spasm is accompanied by slight sweating and tendency to relapse. In these cases, there is a tendency to sleep much, and to suffer from spasms and heaviness in the forehead, while there is also dysuria.

343. Spasms unaccompanied by fever in hysterics are easy to deal with.

344. Spasms unaccompanied by sweating with the production of sputum in a fevered patient are of good significance; in these cases, the onset of relaxed bowels may bring about pyarthrosis.

345. Patients whose eyes are brilliant but with fixed gaze are not in their right mind and they will have a protracted illness.

346. Paroxysms with fits in the manner of a spasm lead to swelling by the ear.

347. In those patients who suffer from trembling and nausea, if slight swellings appear near the ears, the belly being disturbed, it denotes a spasm.

348. Convulsions and tetanus are ended by the supervention of fever.

349. When a convulsion follows a wound, it is a sign of death.

350. When a convulsion supervenes on fever it is a fatal sign; but less so in children.

351. Convulsions do not occur in patients with fever over the age of seven years; if they do occur, it is a fatal sign.

352. A convulsion is ended by the onset of high fever, if there were no fever before, or if there were, a paroxysm of fever. Helpful signs are the passage of much glassy-clear urine, diarrhoea, periods of sleep. Convulsions which occur suddenly are ended by fever or diarrhoea.

353. When a convulsion is attended by prolonged aphasia, it is a bad sign; if such aphasia be short-lived, it is associated either with paralysis of the tongue, or of the arm and right side of the body. The trouble is ended by the sudden passage of a large quantity of urine at one time.

354. Sweats that come on at intervals are beneficial.

355. In tetanus and cases showing opisthotonus, relaxation of the jaws is a sign of death. It is also a sign of death in opisthotonic cases when there is sweating, relaxation of the body, vomiting through the nose, or when aphonia gives way to shouting or to talking nonsense; these things indicate that death will occur on the next day.

356. Opisthotonus accompanied by fever is ended by the passage of urine like semen.

(xix)

357. An anginose condition of the throat which produces no visible sign, either in the neck or in the throat, but which produces intense choking and dyspnoea, proves fatal the same day or on the third day.

358. But those sore throats which cause redness and swellings in the neck, although very similar in most respects, run a longer course.

359. In those cases where there is in addition redness of the throat and of the neck and chest, the sore throat lasts longer and such cases are especially liable to recover unless the redness regress. But if the signs disappear, either without the formation of an external abscess, or without pus being brought up in the mouth mildly and painlessly; and if such does not occur on the critical days, then it is a sign of death. See if an

empyema occurs. The safest thing is for the redness and abscess formation to come to the surface as much as possible.

360. When erysipelas occurs externally, it is a good sign; but if the disease turns inwards, it portends death. This turning internally occurs when the redness disappears, the chest feels heavy and when there is more difficulty in respiration.

361. In cases where sore throats spread to the lung, some patients die within seven days; others survive and form empyemata unless they bring up a quantity of phlegm.

362. If, owing to the violence of the choking, stools are suddenly passed, it is a sign of death.

363. In cases of sore throat without swelling, the production of dry sputum is a bad sign.

364. Swellings on the tongue which accompany a sore throat and which disappear without leaving a trace, are fatal; pains too which depart without obvious cause, are fatal.

365. In cases of sore throat, those who do not quickly spit up ripe sputum are in fatal case.

366. In cases of sore throat, the spread of pains to the head without a sign, in the presence of fever, is fatal.

367. In cases of sore throat, the spread of pains to the legs without a sign, in the presence of fever is fatal.

368. When a sore throat resolves without a crisis occurring, the onset of pain in the hypochondrium with debility and torpor proves unexpectedly fatal, even if the patient appears to be doing well.

369. When a sore throat resolves without a sign, the onset of intense pain in the chest and belly brings about the passage of purulent stools, especially when the illness is ending.

370. Anything supervening in a case of sore throat without producing obvious pain is fatal; long standing pains descend to the legs and there is localization with the formation of an abscess attended with difficulty.

371. Following a sore throat, the violent production of sticky, thick, white sputum is bad and all 'ripening' of this kind is bad. Much purging causes such people to die of paralysis.

372. Following a sore throat, the frequent production of

rather dry sputum with cough and pain in the side, is fatal.
For drinking to provoke a slight cough, or for swallowing to
be forced, is bad.

(xx)

373. Those suffering from pleurisy whose sputum is at the
onset pure pus die on the third day or on the fifth day. If they
survive these days without feeling much better, they begin to
form an empyema on the seventh, ninth or eleventh day.

374. Those suffering from pleurisy who show redness of the
back, whose shoulders are hot, and whose bellies are disturbed
passing bilious foul-smelling stools, are in danger on the
twenty-first day. If they survive this period, they recover.

375. Cases of pleurisy which are dry and in which there is
no sputum are the most difficult; the alarming cases are those
in which the pain is felt high up.

376. Cases of pleurisy attended by rupture of an empyema
are more difficult than those in which this does not occur.

377. Cases of pleurisy in which the tongue becomes bilious
at the beginning, reach a crisis on the seventh day; if this sign
does not occur till the third or fourth day, the crisis will take
place on about the ninth day.

378. If a slightly livid bleb appears on the tongue at the
beginning of the illness, like that formed when red-hot iron is
quenched in oil, resolution is more difficult and the crisis is
reached on the fourteenth day, and they generally spit up
blood.

379. In cases of pleurisy, if ripe sputum be produced by the
third day, resolution is sooner; if it comes later, resolution also
is delayed.

380. In cases of pain due to pleurisy, it is advantageous for
the belly to be soft, the sputum stained; if there be no audible
sounds in the chest, and if the urine run freely. The opposites
of these signs are bad, as also is the sputum becoming sweet.

381. Cases of bilious, and at the same time bloody, pleurisy
generally reach the crisis on the ninth or eleventh day, and
they mostly recover. In cases where the pain is mild at the
beginning, but becomes intense on the fifth or sixth day, the

crisis is more often on the twelfth day and they are not necessarily cured. The greatest danger, in the latter cases, is on the seventh and twelfth days; if they survive twice seven, they recover.

382. Patients with pleurisy whose sputum produces loud râles in the chest, and whose look is downcast, and whose eyes are jaundiced and dim, die.

383. Those who develop empyema following pleurisy, expectorate during the forty days following the bursting.

384. Sputum in all cases of pleurisy and pneumonia should be produced easily and quickly and the yellow matter should be mixed with the sputum; but if the sputum is brought up yellow for a long time after the pain begins, or if it is not mixed and causes much coughing, it is bad. Especially bad is yellow unmixed sputum, the sticky white sputum, the nummular, the green, the frothy, the livid and the rust-coloured. Even worse is that which is so undiluted that it looks dark. If the yellow matter is mixed with a not over-great quantity of blood, this is a sign of recovery if it appears at the beginning of the illness; when it occurs on or after the seventh day, it is less severe. If the sputum is extremely bloody or livid right from the start, it is dangerous. Other bad types are the frothy, the yellow, the dark, the rust-coloured, the sticky and any that quickly becomes coloured. Mucoid or smoky sputum also colours quickly but is a safer sign. Sputa which show the colour associated with ripening within five days of the start of the illness are better.

385. The production of sputum which does not end the pain is bad; if it does, it is useful.

386. Those who bring up both purulent and bilious matter, either separately or mixed together, generally die on the fourteenth day, unless one of the good or bad signs mentioned above supervenes, but failing this they obey the rule. This is especially true when the production of such sputum begins on the seventh day.

387. It is a good thing in these cases, and in all diseases which affect the lungs, for the patient to bear the illness easily, to be free from pain, to bring up sputum easily, to have good

respiration and no thirst, to have the whole body evenly warm and soft, and in addition for sleep, sweating and stools to be good. The reverse is bad. If the production of sputum be attended by all the good signs, the patient will recover; if some of the signs appear but not others, he will not live more than fourteen days; if the contrary signs appear, less than this.

388. All pains in these parts that are not ended either by expectoration, or by venesection and a regimen, end in the formation of empyemata.

389. Those patients recover in whom an abscess forms, following pneumonia, either near the ears or lower down with fistula production. Such abscess formation occurs in cases where both the fever and the pain keep company, in which the sputum does not come according to rule, in which the stools are neither bilious nor loose and unmixed, nor the urine very thick and full of sediment, and in which the other signs indicate probable recovery. Such abscesses occur lower down when there is inflammation in the region of the hypochondrium, in the upper parts when the hypochondrium is slack and painless and bouts of dyspnoea occur for a while and then stop without obvious cause.

390. The formation of abscesses in the legs in dangerous cases of pneumonia is always beneficial; but this is most fortunate when the sputum becomes purulent instead of yellow. If the sputum is not produced normally and the urine does not show a good sediment, there is a risk of the patient becoming lame or, at any rate, of causing a great deal of trouble. If the areas where localization is taking place show retrogression of abscess formation while the fever remains and the sputum fails to appear, there is a risk of the patient becoming delirious and dying. Those patients with pneumonia who are not drained on the proper days, but having had delirium have yet survived the fourteen days, are liable to empyema.

391. Cases of pneumonia which follow pleurisy are safer than those who are pneumonic from the beginning of the illness.

392. Patients of athletic and compact build die more quickly of pleurisy and pneumonia than those of asthenic diathesis.

393. Running at the nose and sneezing are bad signs if they precede or supervene upon an affection of the lungs; in other cases, sneezing is not without benefit.

394. In cases of pneumonia, if the whole tongue becomes covered with rough white fur, both lungs are inflamed; if only half the tongue is affected, only the ipsilateral lung is involved. If the pain is localized near one clavicle only, the upper lobe of one lung is affected; if the pain is in the region of both clavicles, both upper lobes are involved. If the pain is located midway down the side, the middle lobe is affected; if it is near the base, the lower lobe. If there is pain down the whole of one side of the thorax, the whole lung on that side is affected.

If the main bronchi are severely inflamed, so as to rest upon the ribs, there is paralysis of that part of the body and livid patches may appear externally; our predecessors said that such people had had a stroke. If the bronchi are not so severely inflamed as to be in contact, there is general aching all over but no paralysis and no livid patches.

395. In cases where the whole lung is inflamed, together with the heart, so that it is in contact with the ribs, the patient is wholly paralysed and lies cold and insensible. He dies on the second or third day. If this happens without involving the heart, and is not too severe, patients so affected may live longer and sometimes even recover.

396. The formation of empyemata, especially following pleurisy and pneumonia, is attended by pyrexia, slight by day but more intense at night. The patients bring up no sputum worth mentioning, they sweat about the neck and shoulders, their eyes become sunken, the cheeks flushed, the tips of the fingers become warm and rough and the nails become curved; they have fits of chilling, and swelling of the feet, while small blisters appear on the body. They also lose their appetite. These signs appear in chronic empyema. Early rupture is shown by the appearance of certain of these signs early and especially by the early presence of pain and a tendency to dyspnoea. Most empyemata rupture on the twentieth or the fortieth day, or towards the sixtieth. If the pain is intense at the beginning with dyspnoea and a productive cough, expect

the empyema to burst towards the twentieth day or earlier. If the signs are slighter, allow longer in proportion. Calculate the time from the first sign of pain, from the time he had heaviness, or fever, or if ever he had a rigor. Pain, dyspnoea and expectoration must necessarily precede bursting. If the fever goes as soon as rupture has taken place, and the appetite returns, and the pus is brought up easily and is white, odourless, smooth and evenly coloured, and without phlegm, and the stools are small and compact, the patients generally recover quickly. If the fever remains and there is thirst and anorexia, and the pus is livid or greenish, or full of phlegm, or frothy, and the bowels are relaxed, they die. If some of these signs appear, but not all, some patients die; others recover after a long time.

397. Those who are about to develop an empyema bring up sputum which is at first salty, but afterwards becomes sweeter.

398. Those who have tumours in the lungs bring up pus up to forty days after they burst; after this time, they generally become consumptive.

399. A slight epistaxis supervening on pain in the side is a bad sign.

400. In cases of empyema which seem to be recovering, if the sputum continues to have a foul smell, a relapse occurs and proves fatal.

401. Those with pleurisy who, after some time has passed, bring up purulent, somewhat bilious nummular sputum, or purulent and somewhat bloody sputum, are in fatal case. So too are those who expectorate dark sooty matter or sputum resembling dark wine.

402. Those who expectorate frothy blood and have pains in the right hypochondrium, bring it up from the liver; most of them die.

403. Those who, after paracentesis with a hot iron, drain muddy and foul-smelling pus, generally die.

404. Those in whom the pus discolours the probe as would fire, generally die.

405. Patients who suffer from pain in the side, but not of

pleuritic kind, which is accompanied by disturbed, thin favourable stools, turn out to have brain-fever.

406. In diseases of the lungs, a very red epistaxis is bad.

407. Sticky salty sputum associated with hoarseness is bad; following such signs, the appearance of a thoracic swelling is bad; if pains in the neck follow the recession of such a swelling, it is fatal.

408. Hoarseness with cough and relaxed bowels results in the expectoration of pus.

409. In cases of pneumonia, if the urine is thick at the start but becomes thin before four days are up, it is a sign of death.

410. In cases of dry pneumonia, those who bring up a small amount of ripe material cause alarm. If such patients develop somewhat broad red patches on the chest, it is fatal.

411. Pain in the side accompanied by the expectoration of bilious matter which disappears without reason results in ecstasy.

412. Intermittent fever due to an empyema is usually accompanied by slight sweating.

413. The onset of deafness in cases of empyema heralds the passage of bloody stools; towards the end, these people have melaena.

414. A pain in the side accompanied by long continued fever indicates that pus will be brought up.

415. Those who have frequent shivering attacks are on the way to the formation of an empyema; in such a case, a fever may lead to the empyema being formed.

416. In cases where anorexia remains after a pain in the side, and instead there is slight cardalgia, sweating, efflorescence of the complexion, somewhat relaxed bowels, the patient suffers from abscess of the lung.

417. Orthopnoea produces tympanites.

418. The rupture of an empyema is distressing and causes intense pain at the beginning and subsequently, in some cases, leaves discomfort behind. But the most difficult cases are those that occur in the chest, and the danger is especially acute when blood is vomited and when there is much fever and pain about the chest and the broad part of the back. If all these signs are

present, death follows quickly; if not all, and they are not severe, more slowly. The period of inflammation lasts fourteen days at the most.

419. It is best if patients who spit blood are without fever, and cough and ache but slightly, and if the sputum becomes thin after twice seven days. To have fever and cough and intense aching, and always to spit blood which is recent, is not good.

420. In cases where one side shows swelling and is warm, and when it seems as if a weight hangs down when they lie on the other side, the pus is on that side.

421. It is a sign of death when a patient with empyema passes a purulent stool.

422. In wounds of the thorax, if the outside of the wound heals but not the inside, there is a risk of an empyema forming. If the scar on the inside is weak, it may easily burst open.

423. Older people are more likely to die of empyema following pneumonia; younger people die from empyema due to other causes.

424. Those with empyema who, when shaken by the shoulders, make a lot of noise have less pus than those who make but little and who have more difficulty in breathing and a higher colour. Those who make no noise at all and have severe dyspnoea and livid nails, are full of pus and in fatal case.

425. Those who bring up frothy blood, the pain not being below the diaphragm, bring it up from the lungs. If a large blood-vessel in lungs bursts, they eject a large amount of blood and become dangerously ill; if it is a lesser blood-vessel, they bring up less and are more likely to recover.

(xxi)

426. Those with phthisis whose sputum, when thrown on a fire, smells unpleasantly of burnt meat, and who develop alopecia, die.

427. When a patient with phthisis spits into brine and the pus sinks to the bottom, it indicates a speedy death. A bronze vessel should be used to hold the brine.

428. Those with phthisis who develop alopecia die of diarrhoea; when diarrhoea supervenes in phthisis, it is fatal.

429. In diseases like phthisis, suppression of the sputum leads to noisy delirium; in these cases, there is a chance of haemorrhage appearing.

430. The most dangerous cases of phthisis are those where a large blood-vessel ruptures and where there is a catarrhal discharge from the head.

431. The ages between which phthisis is most likely to occur are eighteen to thirty-five years.

432. In cases of phthisis it is bad when itching of the body follows an upset of the bowels.

433. When a gingival discharge accompanied by fever supervenes on a phthisical condition, it is bad.

434. Distension in the hypochondrium is bad in whatever disease it appears, but, among the chronic illnesses, it is worst in phthisis. If it supervenes in cases which show wasting, it is fatal; some have rigors before the end.

435. Eruptions like scratches indicate a wasting condition of the body.

436. In phthisis, those who have a dry dyspnoea, or those who bring up much unripe matter, are in fatal case.

(xxii)

437. Patients suffering from disease of the liver who bring up much bloody sputum, whether it contains either somewhat putrid material or unmixed bilious matter, are likely to die at once.

438. Loss of weight associated with disease of the liver, and accompanied by hoarseness, is bad especially if there is a slight cough.

439. Those with pain in the liver, cardalgia, stupor, rigors, disturbed bowels, loss of weight, anorexia and who have many slight sweats, pass purulent matter in their stools.

440. A sudden pain in the region of the liver is resolved by a fever supervening.

441. Those who spit frothy blood, having a pain in the right hypochondrium, bring it up from the liver, and they die.
S

442 If when the liver has been cauterized, matter like lees of oil comes away, it is a sign of death.

(xxiii)

443. Cases where dropsy develops after an acute disease become painful or end in death. In most cases it first appears in the flanks, though sometimes it starts in the liver. In those cases where it starts from the flanks, the feet swell and long-lasting diarrhoea accompanies the disease, but this diarrhoea neither results in evacuation of the bowels nor does it end pains in the loins and flanks. When the dropsy starts in the liver, it produces an inclination to cough, the feet swell and the stools are hard and produced only after medication; swellings come up in the belly, sometimes on the right and sometimes on the left, and go down again.

444. Strangury supervening on dry dropsy are troublesome; it is also bad when the urine in such cases shows little sediment.

445. Fits supervening on dropsy are a fatal sign, it is also bad when dropsy supervenes on fits, such cases show diarrhoea.

446. In bilious illnesses, disturbance of the belly with the passage of small quantities of material resembling semen and mucus and causing pain in the hypogastrium, and a poor flow of urine; these signs end up in dropsy.

447. If a dropsical patient with fever pass only a small quantity of urine, it is fatal.

448. A watery diarrhoea, without indigestion, supervening on dropsy at its inception, cures the sickness.

449. In cases of dry dropsy, colic arising in the region of the small intestine indicates a poor prognosis.

450. When fits follow dropsy, it is fatal.

451. Dropsy which responds to treatment, but relapses, is hopeless.

452. In cases of dropsy, the draining of fluid from the veins into the belly, brings an end to the condition.

(xxiv)

453. Dysentery which stops at the wrong time causes abscess formation in the ribs, or in the viscera, or in the joints. Is it

bilious dysentery which causes this trouble in the joints; bloody dysentery in the ribs and viscera?

454. In cases of dysentery, the presence of bilious vomiting at the beginning, is bad.

455. In those cases where, after acute dysentery, the fluid (passed) becomes purulent, the supernatant scum is both very white and considerable in amount.

456. The passage of reddish, slimy, copious stools in dysentery, ending with flaming red colours, denotes the risk of madness.

457. In splenetic patients, dysentery is a good sign if it be not too prolonged; but if it is prolonged it is a bad one, for, when it ceases, it is a sign of death if dropsy or diarrhoea occur.

458. In cases of diarrhoea associated with worms, pains which are ended by colic cause swellings around the joints and, following these, the skin becomes red, scaly and blistered. These patients, after slight sweating, turn bright red as if they had been whipped.

459. Patients suffering from prolonged diarrhoea associated with worms, in whom swellings follow the symptoms of colic and pain, have a poor outlook if rigors supervene.

460. Diarrhoea accompanied by dyspnoea ends in phthisis if there is also irritation of the chest.

461. In cases of ileus, vomiting and deafness are bad signs.

(xxv)

462. Hard and painful bladders are always bad, but worst in cases of continued fever; the pain alone which they cause is sufficient to kill the patient; moreover, the bowels do not pass anything in these cases. The condition is terminated by the passage of purulent urine with a smooth white sediment; if it does not end in this way and the bladder does not empty, there is a risk of the patient dying during the first periods of the disease and this is especially likely between the ages of seven and fifteen.

463. Those suffering from stone pass urine easily if they adopt such a posture that the stone does not occlude the urethra. But when dysuria is due to a tumour of the bladder,

difficulty in passing urine is noticed whatever position be adopted. The latter trouble is ended by the discharge of pus.

464. Cases showing incontinence of urine and retraction of the genitalia are hopeless.

465. Ileus supervening on strangury causes death on the seventh day; if not, fever supervenes and a large amount of urine is passed all at once.

(xxvi)

466. Unaccustomed attacks of numbness and anaesthesia are a sign of impending apoplexy.

467. Those who lose the power of movement as the result of wounds are cured if a fever supervenes unattended by a rigor; if such fever does not supervene, they become paralysed on the right side or the left.

468. When haemorrhoids follow apoplexy, it is a good sign; chilling and numbness are bad ones.

469. In cases of apoplexy, sweating supervening on respiratory distress is a sign of death. But if in the same cases, a fever again supervenes, the condition is resolved.

470. Sudden apoplexy accompanied by a low fever is eventually fatal.

471. In cases where some illness terminates in dropsy, where stools are passed resembling the dry pellets of sheep's dung along with mucus, and the urine is not good; there is distension in the hypochondrium and pains and swelling about the belly, and there is pain in the flanks and muscles of the spine. These symptoms are accompanied by fever, thirst and cough. There is dyspnoea on exertion and a heaviness of the legs. Patients who suffer thus go off their food and feel full after eating but little.

472. Diarrhoea puts an end to white oedema. A silent despondency and the avoidance of society is likely to consume patients with this disorder.

473. Delirium with severe chilling following a fright is cured by the onset of fever accompanied by sweating and a good night's sleep.

474. An attack of madness may resolve itself into hoarseness and cough.

475. In cases of madness, a convulsion occurring produces dimness of vision.

476. Cases of silent delirium, with restlessness, a changing gaze, and in which expiration is prolonged, are likely to prove fatal. Such a condition may also result in chronic paralysis or the patients may become insane. Those who have an attack of this sort following upon some abdominal upset pass black stools about the time of the crisis.

477. During the winter, those who, while in health, complain of coldness and heaviness in the loins for only the slightest reason, along with constipation although the upper part of the belly functions well, are likely to suffer from pain in the ischial region, or pain in the kidneys, or the pain of strangury.

478. In cases where there is distress in the region of the lower abdomen, violent irritation having occurred there for some time beforehand, gravel is passed in the urine which tends to be suppressed. In fatal cases of this kind, the mind becomes stupefied.

479. Those who have intensely red superficial blisters about the joints and in whom rigors occur, have their bellies and groins turn bright purplish-red as if with painful blows and die.

480. In cases of jaundice in which the patient is not entirely in control of his senses, the onset of hiccough heralds severe diarrhoea; another possibility is constipation. These patients turn yellowish-green.

481. In cases of pain in the side of the chest which occurs during the course of a fever, and when there is no swelling or other sign, venesection is harmful even if the patient have no appetite and even if the hypochondrium be distended. Bloodletting is also harmful in patients who are not afebrile and who have become sluggish after severe chilling; even though they appear to be the better for it, they die.

(xxvii)

482. It is bad when the head, feet and hands are chilly while the belly and sides are warm; it is best for the whole body to be equally warm and supple.

483. The patient should be easy to move and light when lifted up. Heaviness of the whole body, or of the hands and feet, is bad. If in addition to any heaviness, the fingers and nails become livid, death is at hand. It is a less fatal sign for a part to become black than if it becomes livid. But other considerations should be taken into account; for if the patient is bearing up well, and any of the other good signs appear, the disease is turning to a conclusion, and the parts of the body that have become black, separate.

484. Retraction of the testicles and of the pudendum is a bad sign.

485. It is best for the passage of flatus to be silent; but it is better for its passage to be accompanied by a noise than for it not to be passed at all. However, if wind is passed noisily, it is a bad sign and indicates delirium, unless the patient deliberately emits the wind thus.

486. A wound becoming livid or dry or greenish-yellow, is a sign of death.

487. The best decubitus is that which is customary in health. To lie on the back with the legs stretched out is not a pretty sign, and if the patient slip head first towards the feet, it is worse. It is also a sign of death to have the mouth open and to sleep all the time; or to lie on the back with the legs violently flexed and intertwined. To lie prone, unless this is customary, indicates delirium or pains in the belly. To have the feet and hands uncovered, unless they are extremely hot, and to throw the legs about, is bad as it denotes acute distress. To want to sit up, in acute diseases, is bad, especially in pneumonia and pleurisy. The patient should sleep at night and be awake during the day; the opposite is bad. The least harmful thing is for the patient to sleep from the early morning till the middle of the forenoon; sleep after this is bad. The worst sign is for the patient to sleep neither day nor night, as such insomnia indicates either pain and distress, or delirium.

(xxviii)

488. An incised wound in one temple produces a spasm in the opposite side of the body.

489. If the brain is injured by a blow or in some other way and concussed, the patient immediately falls to the ground, becomes speechless and can neither see nor hear. Most cases are fatal.

490. Following brain injury, fever generally appears and there is bilious vomiting together with paralysis of the body; such patients are in fatal case.

491. The most difficult fractures of the bones of the skull are those which occur along the sutures. Fractures are especially caused by heavy and rounded missiles and, in particular, by those which strike at right-angles, rather than from glancing blows. In order to determine whether there is a fracture present or not, give the patient a stalk of asphodel or fennel to chew with either jaw, and tell him to note whether he notices any bony crepitus; broken bones seem to make a noise.

As time goes on, fractures give rise to signs; sometimes on the seventh day, sometimes on the fourteenth, or at other times. The flesh may come away from the bone which becomes livid; there is pain and fluid collects underneath. It is then difficult to do anything to help.

(xxix)

492. If the omentum prolapses, it inevitably sloughs.

493. If the small intestine be severed, it will not reunite.

494. If a nerve is severed, or the isthmus of the jaw, or the prepuce, the parts will not reunite.

495. If a piece of bone or cartilage in the body be cut off, it will not be replaced by growth.

496. A convulsion following a wound is bad.

497. Bilious vomiting following a wound is bad, especially in head injuries.

498. Injuries to the large nerves generally result in lameness, especially if the wound is oblique and the origins of the muscles, particularly of those in the thighs, are injured.

499. Wounds are most often fatal when they involve the brain, the spinal cord, the liver, the diaphragm, the heart, the bladder, or any of the large blood-vessels. Death also follows any large gashes in the trachea or lungs, so that less air is inspired through the mouth than is lost through the wound. Wounds of the intestine may prove fatal, if the incision is deep and transverse, whether it be the small or large intestine that is involved. If the wound is but small and longitudinal, recovery sometimes occurs. The least fatal wounds are those that affect other parts of the body, or those as far removed as possible from the organs listed above.

500. Dimness of vision occurs in injuries to the brow and in those placed slightly above. It is less noticeable the more recent the wound, but as the scar becomes old, so the dimness increases.

501. The most difficult fistulae are those which occur in the cartilaginous areas and those where there is little fleshy substance, and those which are hollow and which continually burrow and discharge serum, and those where there is a caruncle at the mouth of the fistula. The easiest to treat are those which occur in the soft fleshy places and places free from tendon.

(xxx)

502. The diseases which do not occur before puberty are pneumonia, pleurisy, gout, nephritis, varicose veins of the legs, bloody discharges, cancer unless congenital, white dropsy unless congenital, catarrh of the back, haemorrhoids and ileus of the large bowel unless congenital. None of the above diseases may be expected before puberty. From fourteen to forty-two, the condition of the body is liable to diseases of all kinds. Then again, from that age up to sixty-three, scrofulous swellings in the neck do not occur, neither does stone in the bladder unless it was present previously, nor catarrh of the back, nor nephritis, unless these survive from an earlier age, nor haemorrhoids, nor bloody discharges unless these had occurred before: these diseases are absent up to old age.

(xxxi)

503. A watery discharge before childbirth is bad.

504. Ulceration of the mouth is bad in pregnant women; note whether they suffer from relaxed bowels.

505. Pains which move from the flanks to the small intestine in long illnesses following putrescence of the fœtus and its insufficient discharge, are fatal.

506. Following childbirth or putrescence of the fœtus, a copious and violent lochial discharge which stops, makes for difficulty. A rigor is a bad sign in these cases, as also is disturbance of the belly and especially pain in the hypochondrium.

507. In pregnancy, drowsiness with headache, accompanied by heaviness and convulsions, is generally bad.

508. Those women who, following uterine discharge, have intense pain about the upper part of the belly and in the small intestine, and have diarrhoea and slight nausea—these have attacks of lethargy about the crisis and weakness such as comes from lack of food, and they also have slight sweats and chilling. Relapses occurring in this sort of case prove quickly fatal.

509. Snorting expiration and unaccountable wasting in pregnancy leads to abortion. A pain in the belly after discharge of the fœtus in these cases leads to the discharge of purulent matter.

510. Women who are numbed and whose activity is reduced through weakness, and who are distressed at the crisis with nausea, sweat a great deal. If their bowels are relaxed, it is bad.

511. It is an advantage for a uterine discharge not to be held up; fits may follow such retention, I believe, and in some cases relapse may be prolonged and haemorrhoids supervene.

512. Pain in the hypochondrium is bad in pregnancy; violent diarrhoea and rigor are also of bad significance. Pain in the hypogastrium is less serious if it purges away muddy material; if women who have suffered from this trouble have an early labour they are very ill in the puerperium.

513. Flushing of the face in pregnant consumptives is relieved by the onset of epistaxis.

514. Those women who have white lochia in the puerperium, and in whom cessation of the discharge is attended with a sharp pain in the side with deafness and fever, go into a fatal dementia.

515. Salty (vaginal) discharges during pregnancy indicate trouble due to white pungent lochia during the puerperium; such discharges cause hardness. Hiccough following these signs is bad and so is abnormal contraction of the womb.

516. Rigidity in the feet and loin following uterine discharge leads to suppuration, as also does the painful passage of sticky foul-smelling stools. Choking supervening on the signs mentioned indicates suppuration.

517. A condition in which the womb is both painful and hard is acutely fatal.

518. Painful (vaginal) discharges occurring during pregnancy and associated with aphthous ulceration are of bad significance. The worst sign is the appearance of haemorrhoids.

519. In cases of women suffering from a swollen belly, the spread of redness over the pudendum and the sudden appearance of a white fluid (vaginal) discharge, indicates that they will die following prolonged fever.

520. A spasm is resolved by the onset of menstruation so long as fever does not occur.

521. The presence of rather cloudy matter suspended in the middle of the urine heralds a rigor.

522. A haemorrhage occurring on the fourth day of an illness, indicates that it will be a long one in which the legs will swell and there will be violent diarrhoea.

523. In pregnancy, the onset of drowsy headache with heaviness is bad; such cases are perhaps liable to some sort of fits at the same time.

524. Those women who have pains resembling those of cholera before delivery have an easy labour but take a fever and become very ill, especially if there is any trouble in the

throat, or if any of the signs of bad significance in fever should appear.

525. A 'watery burst' before childbirth is bad.

526. In pregnancy, a salty discharge from the throat is bad.

527. To have a rigor before delivery and then a painless labour is dangerous.

528. A discharge occurring during pregnancy and associated with aphthous ulceration is bad; such patients have a spasm followed by prostration and they become first chilled and then run a high temperature.

529. Snorting expiration during a fever heralds a miscarriage.

530. Shivering, lassitude and heaviness of the head denotes (the onset of) menstruation.

531. Women who are numb to the touch, very dry and without thirst, and who have a copious vaginal discharge, are suffering from a suppurative condition.

532. White lochia appearing suddenly after a miscarriage indicates a difficult course if there is any sign of a rigor, or twitching of the thigh.

533. Aphthous ulceration of the mouth during pregnancy indicates relaxation of the bowels.

534. Delivery in women who are already ill is preceded by rigors.

535. Prostration associated with numbness makes the puerperium a difficult one and causes delirium. Such a condition is not fatal, but it does give previous indication of a copious lochial discharge.

536. When a woman in labour feels pain in the heart, she will shortly expel the child.

537. Shivering, lassitude, heaviness of the head and pain in the neck indicate a violent menstrual flow; when this happens about the time of a crisis and accompanied by a slight cough it means that a rigor will occur.

538. When women who were subject to orthopnoea as girls become pregnant, they suffer from suppuration of the breasts; it is bad if a (vaginal) discharge occurs at the start.

539. Patients who are much disturbed by an acute fever,

and who have pain about the heart but are not bilious, lose the fever if they become maniacal.

540. Haematemesis in multiparous women may help conception.

541. Mistiness of vision is resolved by the onset of a copious menstrual flow.

542. The expectoration of blood which is clotted and not like the lees of wine, in women who have suffered from a fever in which there is pain in the nipples, ends the complaint.

543. Spasms of hysterical nature occurring without fever are easy to manage—as in the case of Dorcas.

544. If a woman has a fatiguing fever after a rigor, a vaginal discharge will start; if the neck is painful in such a case, haemorrhage will occur.

(xxxii)

545. The least harmful sort of vomiting is that in which a mixture of phlegm and bile is brought up, so long as it is of not too great a quantity. The more undiluted the vomit is, the worse it is; green, black or livid vomit is bad. If the same patient vomit matter of all these colours, it is a fatal sign. Livid and foul-smelling vomit indicates the speediest death; red vomit is also a sign of death, especially if it is brought up with painful straining.

546. Intense nausea which does not result in vomiting is bad; so also is intense and unproductive retching.

547. Small quantities of bilious vomit are bad, especially if accompanied by insomnia.

548. Deafness supervening on the vomiting of a small quantity of dark material does no harm.

549. The repeated vomiting of bilious and undiluted matter at short intervals is bad when associated with severe distress and intense pain in the loins.

550. Nausea, a twanging voice and an appearance of the eyes as if they were covered with wool, when following vomiting, is a sign of madness. Patients who suffer thus die with aphonia after an acute spell of dementia.

551. It is a bad sign for someone who is thirsty to vomit and subsequently to lose his thirst.

552. In cases where nausea accompanies insomnia, parotid swellings are especially likely to occur.

553. In cases of nausea in which an upset of the bowels is followed by constipation, an eruption resembling mosquito bites quickly appears and a lachrymose discharge occurs from the eyes.

554. Hiccough following the vomiting of undiluted material is bad; a spasm is bad too. It is much the same in cases of over-purging due to the administration of drugs.

555. Those about to vomit, spit first.

556. A convulsion following the administration of hellebore is fatal.

557. In every case of excessive purging, it is fatal for the patient to break out in a cold sweat. It is bad in these cases if the patients vomit repeatedly and feel thirsty. If there is nausea and pain in the loins, the bowels are relaxed.

558. Evacuation of very dark red material due to the administration of hellebore is bad; prostration following this is bad.

559. It is beneficial to vomit small amounts of red frothy material after a dose of hellebore; it causes hardness and resolves large areas of suppuration. Those who produce a vomit of this kind are specially liable to pains in the chest, to slight sweats during rigors, and to swelling of the testicles. Once this complication has occurred, a rigor follows and the swelling goes down.

560. Frequently repeated attacks of vomiting with the same symptoms leads to the production of dark vomit about the time of the crisis, and patients who suffer so also show twitching.

(xxxiii)

561. The best kind of sweating is that which brings a fever to an end on a critical day; it is useful too if sweating relieves a fever. Cold sweating confined to the head and neck is of poor significance because it denotes a long and dangerous illness.

562. Cold sweating is a sign of death in a high fever; of prolonged illness in a milder one.

563. Sweating appearing at the same time as fever in an acute disease is of bad significance.

(xxxiv)

564. In fever, urine which shows a white smooth sediment on standing denotes rapid resolution of the disease; of similar significance is urine which contains poorly separated fatty material. Pink urine, and that which has a smooth pink sediment, appearing before the seventh day of the disease, indicates resolution on the seventh day; if such urine appears after the seventh day, the disease will end later on. If on the fourth day the urine has a pink cloud in it, resolution will occur on the seventh day so long as the other symptoms are in accord. Urine which is thin and bilious and which has a slightly sticky sediment, and that which shows fluctuations, indicates a chronic illness. If this latter sort of urine is passed for long, or if the urine becomes worse about the time of the crisis, the case is not without danger.

565. Watery and white urine throughout in chronic cases means that there will be difficulty in attaining a crisis, while recovery is uncertain.

566. Clouds in the urine, if white and low, are beneficial; if they are red or dark or livid, they indicate a difficult illness.

567. Dangerous kinds of urine are those which are bilious looking but not pink in acute diseases, those like barley-meal with a white sediment, and those which vary both as to colour and sediment—especially in cases who have catarrh of the head. Other dangerous signs are for the urine to change from a dark colour to a thin and bilious appearance, for urine which has produced sediment to change to one in which the material is dispersed, and for urine which has been turbid to produce a livid muddy sediment. Note whether pain in the hypochondrium—the right one, I think—follows such signs, or whether the patients become jaundiced and have pain in the region of the ear. If such patients have violent diarrhoea shortly afterward, it is fatal.

568. It is a bad sign when urine suddenly becomes 'ripe' for a short while contrary to expectations; generally speaking, any unexpected ripening in an acute disease is a poor sign. It is also bad if such signs are followed by an intensely red eruption, the spots being covered with a rust-coloured scab. The passage of colourless transparent urine is bad; it is seen specially in brain-fever. It is also bad when urine is passed soon after drinking, especially in pleurisy and pneumonia. Oily urine passed before a rigor is also bad. Another bad sign in acute diseases is the appearance of greenish streaks below the surface.

569. Fatal signs in the urine are for it to be dark or to have a dark sediment. In children, thin urine is of more fatal significance than thick, but the reverse is true in the case of the thin. The passage of urine, which in cases of distortion appears to contain particles like hailstones, is painful. Urinary incontinence is fatal. In pneumonia, it is fatal if the urine, being ripe at the beginning, becomes thin after the fourth day.

570. In cases of pleurisy, the passage of dusky and bloody urine containing a variable amount of sediment which does not settle, generally leads to a fatal issue within fourteen days. Green urine containing a dark or bran-like sediment also denotes a rapid death in cases of pleurisy. In cases of *causus* associated with fits, the urine of worst significance is the very white kind.

571. The persistence of 'raw' urine longer than it should be passed, while the other signs betoken recovery, denotes abscess formation and pain, especially in the infra-diaphragmatic regions. If there are wandering pains in the loins, abscess formation will be localized in the hip, whether fever be present or not. Fatty urine with a sediment indicates fever; bloody urine passed at the beginning of an illness denotes that it will be a lengthy one. When disturbed urine accompanies sweating, it means a relapse will take place. White urine like that of cattle indicates headache; that with a membrane in it, a convulsion. Urine with a sediment in it resembling sputum, or muddy slime, indicates a rigor. Cobwebby urine denotes wasting. In irregular fevers, dark cloudlets in the urine herald

a quartan. Colourless urine with dark matter in suspension, accompanied by insomnia and distress, indicates brain-fever. Ash-coloured urine accompanied by dyspnoea indicates a dropsical complaint.

572. Watery urine, or that which is turbid with friable particles, indicates the onset of diarrhoea. Does very white urine becoming, as it were, full of hairs, indicate future sweating? And does froth on the surface of urine, indicate that sweating has occurred?

573. In tertian fevers with shivering, things like dark cloudlets in the urine denote that the shivering is irregular. Urine with membranes in it, and urine passed with shivering and forming a sediment, denote a convulsion.

574. Urine which has shown a favourable sediment and suddenly loses it denotes distress and change. Urine which settles after stirring denotes that a rigor will occur about the time of the crisis and possibly also a change to a fever of quartan or tertian periodicity.

575. In cases of pleurisy, pink coloured urine with a smooth sediment denotes a safe crisis. Urine of a bright yellow colour with a white sediment means that the crisis will not only be safe but come quickly. Urine of a bright red colour with a well-demarcated smooth yellow sediment denotes a long and distressing illness with complications, but one which will not end fatally. White watery urine with a light brown sediment like barley-meal denotes both a distressing course and danger. Yellow urine with a light brown sediment like barley-meal denotes a long and dangerous illness.

576. In cases of parotid swellings, it is a bad sign if the urine quickly and for a short time becomes 'ripe'. For the patient to become thoroughly chilled in these circumstances is bad.

577. Stoppage of the bladder, especially when associated with headache, suggests that convulsions will occur; numbness with prostration in such a condition is difficult but not fatal; note whether there be any sign of delirium.

578. Sudden renal pain with retention of urine indicates the passage of small stones or of inspissated urine. Twitching and

fever appearing in such circumstances in older people is also sometimes a sign of the passage of small stones.

579. Retention of urine and heaviness in the abdomen is generally a sign of the onset of strangury; if not, of some other disease to which the patient has previously been subject.

580. In bilious diseases, suppression of urine leads to a quick death.

581. In the course of a fever, the appearance of urine containing suspended hairy fragments denotes either a relapse or a sweat.

582. In protracted slight irregular fevers, the passage of thin urine denotes disease of the spleen.

583. In a fever, the passage of urine of different sorts at different times denotes a long illness.

584. Urine which is passed only when the patients are reminded to urinate is specially fatal in its significance; note whether such patients pass urine which looks as if its sediment had been stirred up.

585. In cases where the urine is scanty and contains clots, the patient not being afebrile, the subsequent passage of a copious amount of thin urine is beneficial. This occurs when a urinary sediment has been present either from the beginning, or shortly after the beginning, of the illness.

586. If the urine soon shows the appearance of a sediment, the crisis will be reached quickly.

587. In cases of epilepsy, the appearance of thin and unripe urine contrary to what is usual, and not due to over-eating, denotes a fit. This is specially true if there is pain in the acromial region, or in the neck and back, or if there is a convulsion, or numbness of the body, or if the patient has a troubled dream.

588. Anything which comes in small quantities, such as a small epistaxis, or scanty urine, or scanty vomit or stools, is always bad. This is particularly true if any of these signs are closely associated.

(xxxv)

589. The best sort of stool is that which is soft, compact, rather reddish-brown, not specially foul-smelling, and which

T

is passed at the same accustomed time. Its size should be in accord with the amount of food taken and the stools should become thick towards the time of the crisis. It is also beneficial if round worms are ejected at the approach of the crisis.

590. In acute diseases, a frothy and very bilious stool is bad; so too is a very white one and, even worse, is a mealy dung-like stool. Stupor following such signs is bad; so also is the passage of bloody material and unexplained inanition.

591. In cases where there is constipation with only the forced passage of small dark stools like the dung of sheep and goats, a copious epistaxis is bad.

592. A sticky, unmixed, or white stool is of poor significance; so too is one which is densely packed and fermented and which somewhat resembles mucus. A somewhat livid purulent sediment with bilious matter formed from turbid stools is also bad.

593. To pass bright red blood in the stools is bad, especially if there is any pain present.

594. A frothy, very bilious stool is bad; jaundice may follow.

595. A frothy efflorescence on bilious stools is bad, especially if the patient has a pain in the loins or is doubled-up. The aching pains in such cases are intermittent.

596. A thin frothy stool with a watery sediment is bad; so too is a purulent one. A dark and bloody stool is of bad significance during the course of a fever and in certain other circumstances. A variegated stool of full colour is poor, and the worse the more alarming its colour. However, an exception may be made when a purge has been administered, in which case such an appearance is not dangerous so long as the stool is only of moderate size. A soft friable stool is of poor significance in fever; so too is a dry friable discoloured one, especially if the bowels are relaxed; if dark stools have preceded this, the sign is fatal.

597. Copious liquid stools passed at short intervals are bad, for they may sometimes cause insomnia, sometimes prostration.

598. A moist somewhat friable stool associated with chilling

in patients who are not apyrexial, is poor; rigors following this cause suppression of urine and of faeces.

599. The passage of very watery stools which does not stop in acute illnesses is bad, especially if the patient does not complain of thirst.

600. A very red thin stool is poor; so too is one which is particularly yellow, or white, or frothy, or watery. A small sticky stool and a smooth yellowish one are also bad. A fluid stool is of most serious significance in patients with coma or in those who are numb. It is a sign of death to have a haemorrhage containing many clots of blood; so too is a white fluid stool associated with abdominal distension.

601. A dark stool like blood is bad whether the patient be febrile or not; so too are all variegated stools and those of a very intense colour.

602. Stools which end in the passage of frothy unmixed material, denote the onset of a paroxysm in all cases but especially in patients suffering from convulsions; parotid swellings may follow. The passage of stools which become fluid and then solid again, being unmixed and like manure, denotes a long illness. A very red stool in a fever denotes delirium. A white faecal stool passed by a jaundiced patient denotes a difficult illness, so too does a fluid stool which takes on a red hue on starting in cases of haemorrhage.

603. A sticky stool variegated with dark patches is bad, especially when the stools are very white ones.

604. A very white stool in the course of a fever means that the crisis will not be reached easily.

605. Disturbance of the bowels with frequent desire to go to stool, but the passage of very little, causes trismus. It is ended if the face becomes suffused.

606. Faeculent stools passed with straining denotes a bad condition of the intestine; the passage of mucous stools in acute illnesses with pain in the region of the heart, denotes dysentery and perhaps pain in the loins. In such cases, a general tension of the abdomen and the forced passage of fluid stools while the belly quickly becomes puffed out, give

rise to suspicion that convulsions will occur. When a rigor supervenes in such cases, it is fatal.

607. Those who pass dark stools have slight cold sweats.

608. In cases where the bowels are disordered from the start of the illness and the urine is scanty, and, as time passes, the stools become normal and the urine comes in good quantity but is thin, localization will occur in the joints.

609. Frequent going to stool provokes rigors; when the stool is of poor significance this denotes most difficulty when it begins on the fourth day of the disease.

610. Frequent going to stool at short intervals, the stools being rather sticky and containing small amounts of faecal matter, with pain in the hypochondrium and the side, indicates the onset of jaundice. Note whether, when such stools stop, the patients turn yellow. I think that such patients also suffer from haemorrhage. Pains in the loins in these cases indicate haemorrhage.

611. If bright red blood is passed with stupor and headache, it is fatal for the patient to become pyrexial.

612. Sticky bilious stools are especially likely to result in parotid abscess.

613. Any swellings that come up with pain in patients with relaxed bowels, are bad. When the bowels become constipated, provided no new factor emerges, such swellings quickly burst and this is of worse significance. The vomit in such cases is bad and offensive.

614. In cases where inflamed and very red stools cease and are replaced by foul-smelling, copious reddish ones, there is a risk of dementia.

615. A parched skin indicates a disordered state of the belly; in such cases, very red stools and stools containing purulent fleshy matter are especially likely to be passed.

616. Following the passage of soft faeculent stools, the appearance of coma results in parotid swellings.

617. Deafness puts an end to bilious stools, and a bilious stool puts an end to deafness.

618. Herpetic eruptions, above the level of the groin, which extend to the flank and pubis indicate a bad state of the belly.

619. Prostration which cures pain is specially likely to result in diarrhoea.

620. Painful suppurating ulcers in the anal region causes an upset of the bowels.

621. Types of stool which indicate death are: the greasy, the dark, livid stools with a foul smell, bilious stools which contain matter like pounded lentils or chick-peas or like clots of bright-coloured blood and in smell resembling those of infants, and the variegated. A stool of the last kind may also indicate a chronic illness, and a stool of this sort may also be bloody, full of scrapings, bilious, dark, green, either all at the same time or successively. Incontinence of faeces is also a sign of death.

622. Difficulty in swallowing fluid, with tussive respiration, belching stifled and muffled, denotes abdominal distress.

623. Also bad are very red stools occurring on the fourth day of an illness, and such haemorrhages lead to coma. After these signs, the patients die in convulsions having first passed dark stools.

624. Those who pass dark stools have slight cold sweats.

625. Sudden unexplained prostration of the bowels in chronic patients with wasting, accompanied at the same time by aphonia and twitching, are fatal. Thin stools of dark matter passed with shivering are better for such patients and stools of this latter kind are particularly beneficial in the years before full adult age is reached.

626. In all cases, irritation indicates the passage of dark stools and the vomiting of clots. Twitching with gnawing pain and headache denotes the passage of dark stools. Previously matter resembling vomit is passed, and if vomiting occurs, much matter of a similar nature is also brought away.

627. When following a disturbance of the bowels, the symptoms become more pronounced about the crisis, dark stools are passed.

628. Following prolonged diarrhoea with vomiting, biliousness and anorexia, a profuse sweat with sudden weakness is fatal.

629. When copious thin blood is seen in liquid stools as a result of purging, it is a poor sign.

630. Rigidity of the belly, associated with pain and accompanied by shivering and fever with anorexia, leads to the formation of collections of pus if the belly subsequently becomes somewhat relaxed but insufficiently so as to produce purging.

631. Disturbance of the bowels with the passage of acrid stools never occurs in coma and stupor.

632. Following relaxed bowels, lassitude, headache, thirst, insomnia and, when these symptoms are ended, with a suffused complexion, there is a risk of dementia.

633. If a patient suffers from dyspnoea, should he become yellow, his respiration improves and he loses his appetite, the bowels then being opened.

634. Scalding stools passed with tenesmus, denote a disturbed state of the belly.

635. In the bilious, disturbed bowels with the frequent passage of small stools containing mucus associated with tenesmus, lead to pain in the region of the small gut. The urine then not being passed freely, such cases end in dropsy.

636. A tremulous tongue is sometimes a sign of impending diarrhoea.

637. When a patient has high pyrexia, the passage of frothy stools accompanies a paroxysm of the fever.

638. Following relaxation of the bowels, chilling associated with sweating is a poor sign.

639. Following relaxation of the bowels, haemorrhage from the gums is a sign of death.

640. A pure stool supervening, an acute fever reaches its termination with sweating.

GENERAL INDEX

A

Abdomen (*see also* Belly)
  distension of, 78, 80, 159, 246, 275
  distress in, 261
  enlargement of, 77
  haemorrhage into, 170
  pain in, 114, 164, 174
  tension in, 275
Abdominal tumour, 232
Abortion (*see* Miscarriage)
  procuration of, 9
  threatened, 167
Abscess, 64, 92, 162, 228, 230, 245, 249
  critical, 35
  formation of, 34
  gingival, 231, 237
  hepatic, 28
  of joints, 125, 228, 258
  of legs, 122, 252
  of lung, 255
  of neck, 248
  parotid (*see also* Parotid swellings),
    122, 228, 242, 276
  peri-anal, 55
  perineal, 32
  retro-pharyngeal, 157
  of shoulders, 171
  subdiaphragmatic, 28
  of teeth, 64
  types of, 116
  urethral, 164
Acromium, pain in, 221, 273
Adenitis, cervical, 157
Agitation, 71
Ague, 91
Alopœcia in phthisis, 256
Amazons, 104
Ambidexterity, 175
Amenorrhoea, 168
Anaesthesia, 260
Anatomy of blood-vessels, 209, 210
  functional significance of, 22
Angina of throat, 248
Anorexia, 63, 66, 173, 223, 232, 243,
  244, 255, 257
Anuria, 45, 172, 240
Anus, blood-vessels to, 210
  pain in, 59, 71, 223
  ulceration of, 165, 277
Aorta, tumours near, 212

Anxiety, 190
Aphasia, 71, 221, 248
Aphonia, 71, 79, 185, 238, 244, 247,
  248, 268, 277
  with dementia, 239
  in epilepsy, 188
  rigors with, 239
Aphorisms, 148
Aphthae, 63, 65, 157
Aphthous ulceration, 266, 267
Apnoea in epilepsy, 188
Apollo, 198
Apollo Nomius, 182
Apoplexy, 154, 156, 157, 158, 173,
  230, 260
  haemorrhoids in, 260
Appetite, loss of, 34, 169
Arcturus, 100, 101
  rising of, 8, 32, 36, 63
Arm, erysipelas of, 64
  paralysis of, 53, 248
  blood-vessels of, 210
Arthritis, 156, 157, 158
Ascaris (*see also* Worms), 157, 231, 247
Ascites, 158, 176
Asia, character of, 101
Asiatics, qualities of, 102, 109
Asthenia, 220
Asthma, 91, 132, 157, 158, 184, 185
  kyphosis in, 172
Astronomy, importance in medicine
  of, 91
Athena, 198
Athletes, health of, 148
Athletic constitution, 211
Athletics, diet for, 15
Aura in epilepsy, 189
Auricles, 192
Axis vertebra, 240
Azov, sea of, 103

B

Back, pain in, 210, 223, 240, 244, 260,
  273
Baldness in eunuchs, 171
  with varicose veins, 171
Barbarians, 102
Barley-cake, 208
Barley-gruel, qualities of, 130
Barley-meal, 137

279

U

SUPPLEMENTARY INDEX

THIS index lists certain morbid conditions which, although not necessarily mentioned by name in the text, are certainly, probably, or possibly described therein. The index should be used in conjunction with the General Index.

In giving references the following abbreviations are used:

TM	=	Tradition in Medicine
E(I)	=	Epidemics, Book I
E(III)	=	Epidemics, Book III
SM	=	Science of Medicine
AWP	=	Airs, Waters, Places
P	=	Prognosis
A	=	Aphorisms
SD	=	The Sacred Disease
CP	=	Coan Prognosis

Where a cross reference is marked with an asterisk (*) the subject will be found in the General Index.

A

	Reference	*Page*
Abortion, incomplete	CP, xxxi, 505	265
,, ,,	CP, xxxi, 506	265
,, septic	CP, xxxi, 509	265
Abscess, apical	CP, viii, 232	238
,, cervical	CP, xix, 359	248
,, hepatic (*see* Amœbiasis, hepatic)		
,, perinephric	A, VII, 36	174
,, pulmonary	A, IV, 47	161
,, pulmonary	CP, xx, 400	254
,, retro-pharyngeal	CP, xiv, 261	240
,, subdiaphragmatic	A, VII, 54	176
,, ,,	TM, 22	28
Acquired characteristics, inheritance of	AWP, 14	103
Adenitis, tuberculous	A, III, 26	157
,, ,,	CP, xxx, 502	264
Allergy	TM, 20	25
Amœbiasis, hepatic	E(III), 17, case xiii	77
,, ,,	P, 7	116
,, ,,	CP, xx, 402	254
,, ,,	CP, xxii, 437	257
,, ,,	CP, xxii, 439	257
,, ,,	CP, xxii, 441	257
,, ,,	CP, xxii, 442	258
,, pulmonary	CP, xx, 402	254
,, ,,	CP, xxii, 437	257
,, ,,	CP, xxii, 442	258
Anaemia in children	CP, xvii, 333	246
Angina pectoris	CP, xv, 280	242
Appetite, perversion of	CP, xvii, 333	246
Arteriosclerosis, cerebral	CP, iv, 157	230
,, ,,	CP, xxvi, 466	260
Aura in epilepsy	SD, 15	189
Automatism, post epileptic	SD, 1	179